THE

DNA

ADVANTAGE

By Patty Lach Daigle

Edited by Lil Barcaski

Published by: GWN Publishing
www.GWNPublishing.com

Cover Design: Kristina Conatser

ISBN: 978-1-959608-81-3

This book is dedicated to those who GOD put in my path to help heal me.

TESTIMONIALS

You are so thoughtful when it comes to a hard to please customer. You are always there to refer me to the best vitamins and products. I trust your advice. Love,

—T. CLAVET

Patty Daigle has been a pivotal factor in helping me realize the value of DNA testing. I am 78 years old and have been living in pain the majority of my life. Patty helped me focus on myself and how DNA testing could change my life with the knowledge that I learned from her and the Ütrition specifically formulated for my DNA results. Patty took the time to help me understand the results and to assist me with any questions that were difficult for me to understand. No matter how busy she is or where she is, Patty is always available to help me gain optimal health through the DNA results. She is very knowledgeable in all health wellness areas. Thank you, Patty Daigle.

—C. WILLIAMS

The DNA test started this quest of finding out more about my internal footprint. Identifying areas that needed some attention, some boost! Greens Caps have lowered my blood pressure; BP that I have not had in years. Booster caps have increased my energy along with better sleep since taking them daily. Patty is a great resource, keeping me informed and on track!

—A. KROLL

My name is Noah. I'm a past Barcelona Academy soccer player and I've encountered kind of a problem where I have been injured over the past 4 years and I have been always missing the vital nutrients that I needed, I never knew what it was. But after sending in my DNA lab work that I sent in through the mail, they were able to customize my own nutrition for me, and I've only been using it for about a little over 6 months now, but the results have been amazing. And I haven't been injured since. My body finally feels like it was before I was injured and I would definitely recommend it for any further athletes that are trying to stay fit and stay healthy and get back in touch with how they played in their prime in any sport. Because everyone is lacking in vitamins in some area or another, and I couldn't be more grateful for the outcome that I've experienced so far.

—N. MARTIN

We really don't realize what it takes for our bodies to function right or what we are missing until we take a test and see what is going on inside of us and what we need to function right. After being tested I was amazed at what was going on inside of me and what my body was missing. So then my new health journey started. I began taking Utrition vitamins made just for me. What a big change it has made in my health. I have noticed my body doesn't hurt the way it used to, I have more energy and I am able to get out and do more of the things I used to and not have to worry about how much I am going to hurt the next day. Utrition has helped me so much health wise and has given me back part of my life that I was missing.

This product can help you out so much and help your body get back on track to start functioning so much better. I would highly recommend you to at least try this product out. You will be amazed at how much better your body is going to respond and how much better you are going to feel.

—S. COLON

TABLE OF CONTENTS

INTRODUCTION

Welcome to a journey towards achieving personal wellness like never before. In this book, we'll explore two fascinating areas of science—Epigenetics and Nutritional Genomics—that are shaping the future of health and nutrition.

Allow me to simplify what might seem like complex concepts:

Epigenetics is all about how your behavior and environment can change the way your genes work. Unlike changes to your actual DNA—your genetic code—these changes are like dimmer switches on a light, turning gene activity up or down based on external factors. So, the food you eat, the stress you feel, and even the air you breathe can all influence your genes and, consequently, your health.

Nutritional Genomics, or "nutrigenomics" for short, zooms in even further. It studies how different foods can affect your genes. For example, some foods might turn certain genes on or off, directly impacting how you process nutrients and maintain health. This means what you eat can be tailored specifically to your own genetic makeup, potentially leading to better health outcomes.

So, why focus on one and not the other? Well, depending on your specific health concerns or wellness goals, one approach might tell you more about what you need for your body to find balance and thrive.

This book is your invitation to understand how unique you are, right down to your DNA, and how that uniqueness can guide your choices for a healthier life. Forget one-size-fits-all health advice—it's time to learn how your body works on a genetic level and protect yourself against illnesses in a way that's tailored just for you.

Get ready to unlock the secrets within your DNA and step into the future of well-being.

> Embark with me on an exciting journey of
> self-discovery and targeted wellness where you no
> longer have to guess which health advice suits you—
> science can help pinpoint it for you.

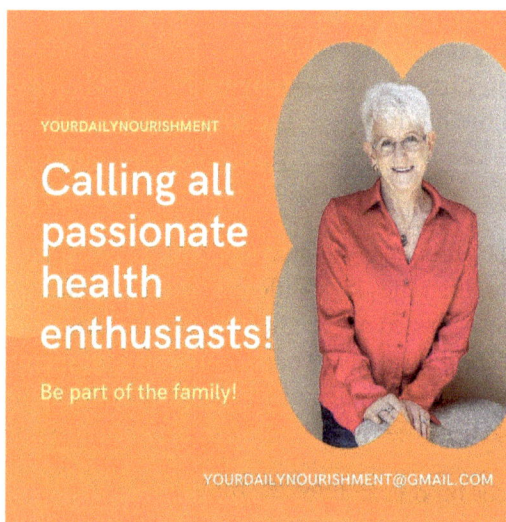

PREFACE

How did DNA passion come into play?

My journey into the world of DNA testing began with a simple curiosity about my heritage. Growing up, I knew very little about my family history beyond a few stories about my grandparents who were from Poland. But as I delved deeper into genealogy research and DNA analysis, I started to uncover connections and details about my ancestors that I never knew existed. I will share a little more below.

In 2019, I was in major health decline. I was feeling lethargic, lost 30 pounds in six months, and my immune system was shutting down. With no success from the medical doctors in figuring out the problem, a friend of mine suggested epigenetic testing. More about this in Chapter 2. Little did I know I would learn so much more about the needs of my body.

Despite the excitement of discovering my roots, there was one aspect of my DNA test results that initially shocked and saddened me: the presence of certain genetic variants associated with pregnancy loss.

As someone who had struggled with infertility and multiple miscarriages, this information hit close to home. It was difficult to accept that my own genetic makeup may have played a role in my reproductive struggles. During the first year and a half of being married, I lost three pregnancies. For twenty-nine years I wondered why? This was an emotional and physical strain on me for many years. I found through the testing that certain genes that I carry may have been the cause for these losses.

As I continued to educate myself on genetics and fertility, I began to understand that it wasn't just about blaming my genes for past losses. Instead, knowing about these variants gave me insight into potential health risks and allowed me to make informed decisions about family planning and to share with my daughter.

Having this information prompted me to be more proactive about my overall health. I made changes to my diet, exercise routine, and stress management techniques in order to optimize my chances for a healthy lifespan. And even though there are no guarantees when it comes to reproductive health (especially being over 60), I felt empowered knowing that I was taking charge of my own well-being.

I wanted to start sharing the knowledge I have gained and help others with their own DNA journeys. How it affects every aspect of life—from relationships to health to culture. The book offers practical advice on how to use genetic information responsibly; and explores the potential of DNA testing to empower individuals and families.

I hope this book will be a source of comfort, inspiration, and guidance for those who are grappling with similar challenges and seeking to make sense of their health and new reality. I hope to provide clarity on complex topics such as genetic testing, getting your life back, carrier screening, medical research, and privacy in the digital age.

DNA is the foundation of who you are, and understanding it can help you make informed decisions about your health. Whether you're dealing with a genetic predisposition, facing a difficult medical diagnosis, or simply curious about your family health, this book will give you the tools to navigate the world of nutritional genomics with confidence and empowerment. Through my own experiences, I highlight the importance of open communication within families when it comes to discussing genetic information and making informed decisions.

I will touch on topics such as genetic markers and ethical considerations in DNA testing, and how to understand your genetic code and interpret it in ways that are meaningful to you. With this knowledge, you can make sensible decisions backed by science and data. From what foods to eat, supplements and vitamins that may be good for you, how much exercise is right, and more— knowing your genetics gives you a powerful tool in understanding your health.

I never even knew epigenetics existed. With each new story, I am discovering more and more about myself and my family's health. I am so grateful for this exciting adventure of discovery – one that has been filled with surprises and new information about my personal history. It's a journey unlike any other – one that is helping me to learn so much more about who I am that I never could have found out on my own.

I hope to use this knowledge to not only deepen my understanding of myself, but also to inspire those around me. We all have our own unique stories to tell and by exploring our family histories, we can gain a greater appreciation for who we are. Plus, it's a great way to connect with your loved ones.

With these chapters of guidance, you will have all the tools needed to make health and wellness part of your everyday life. By learning how to regulate stress, create a balanced lifestyle and prioritize your health, you'll be on your way to living a life of abundance, joy and positivity.

So dive in and start your journey! There is no better time than today to begin taking the steps towards a healthier and happier you. With dedication and perseverance, anything is possible. Let's get started!

Good luck!

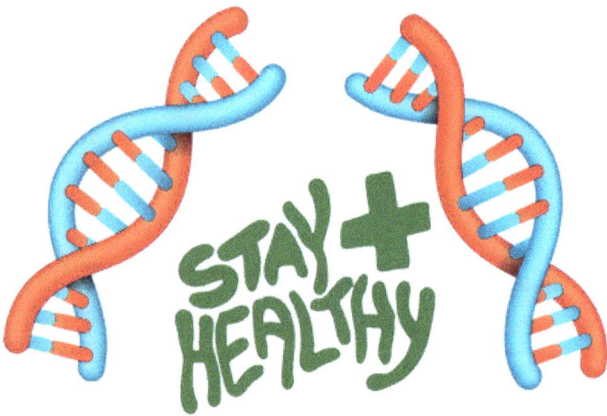

STAY + HEALTHY

The importance of addressing DNA Health

CHAPTER 1

WHY ADDRESS DNA?

I t is the empowerment you can gain from knowing about your-self from the inside out. What if you could unlock the mystery of why your body reacts in different ways to different diets, medications, or environmental triggers?

First, I must explain the reasons for addressing DNA with you. It is about DNA health; nutritional genomics and epigenetics. You see, your genetic make-up is made up of a combination of your parents' DNA profiles, and this particular combination can be used to determine risks for certain diseases or health issues. Knowing which genes in your DNA are most affected by diet, lifestyle and environment can help you personalize how you prevent, manage and monitor various health conditions. The information gleaned from a comprehensive DNA analysis can give you a better under-standing of your individual health needs and how best to go about meeting those needs.

From biomarker tests, researchers are able to identify your unique genetic markers that indicate an increased risk for certain diseases or conditions. This is where the DNA Advantage comes in. We use this knowledge to create personalized nutrition plans and lifestyle adjustments tailored specifically to each individual user. With the right nutrition and lifestyle choices, you can lower your risk for many health issues. With comprehensive DNA analysis services, we will help you identify which health risks you may be more susceptible to so that you can take proactive measures to improve your overall health status.

My goal is to provide you with as much information as possible and empower you to take control of your health. With The DNA Advantage, you can learn more about yourself and your risks for certain diseases or conditions, allowing you to make lifestyle adjustments that will improve your overall health status. Where your personalized nutrition plans are designed to help you optimize your diet according to your specific needs, and our lifestyle advice will help guide you in making choices that promote health and wellbeing.

Cultivating healthy habits is now my path to optimal well-being.

In today's fast-paced world, it's easy to overlook the importance of maintaining good health. However, our habits play a significant role in shaping our overall well-being. Through trial and error, I have discovered a set of habits that have helped me prioritize my health and achieve a state of optimal well-being. Here are a few personal habits that have positively impacted my physical and mental health.

1. REGULAR EXERCISE:

Physical activity is the cornerstone of a healthy lifestyle. I make it a point to engage in regular exercise, whether it's a brisk walk, a workout at the gym, or a yoga session. Exercise not only helps me stay physically fit but also boosts my mood, reduces stress, and enhances my overall productivity.

2. BALANCED DIET:

Maintaining a balanced diet is vital for nourishing the body and mind. I focus on consuming a variety of fresh fruits, vegetables, whole grains, lean proteins, and healthy fats. I prioritize nutrient-dense foods, avoiding excessive processed or sugary items and flour. Additionally, I practice portion control and mindful eating to ensure I am fueling my body adequately.

3. HYDRATION:

Drinking sufficient water is often underestimated, but it is a habit that has transformative effects on our health. I ensure I stay hydrated throughout the day by carrying a water bottle with me at all times. Proper hydration helps regulate body temperature, supports digestion, improves cognitive function, and boosts overall energy levels. Unlock the power of hydration: the secret to vitality and well-being. Discover the incredible benefits of drinking enough water, a simple habit with profound effects on your health. Stay effortlessly hydrated all day long by keeping a trusty water bottle by your side. Experience the transformative effects of proper hydration: regulate body temperature, enhance digestion, sharpen cognitive function, and supercharge your energy levels. Take it to the next level with hydrogenated water. Quench your thirst and unleash your full potential.

1. **CLEANSING AND DETOXIFICATION:** Drinking hydrogenated water helps flush toxins out of the body by entering cells and binding to heavy metals and impurities to make them water soluble so the body can easily expel them. This promotes detoxification and cleansing.

2. **BOOSTS ENERGY LEVELS:** Hydrogen helps reduce lactic acid in muscles which prevents fatigue. Drinking hydrogen water can increase metabolic efficiency and endurance.

3. **ANTI-AGING BENEFITS:** Hydrogen may protect cells from oxidative stress which slows the aging process. It fights free radical damage to keep skin looking youthful.

4. **SUPPORTS HEART HEALTH:** Hydrogen acts as an antioxidant to prevent damage to LDL cholesterol which may lower heart disease risk. It also reduces inflammation which is linked to heart attacks and strokes.

5. **GUT HEALTH AND IMMUNITY:** Hydrogen water helps maintain a healthy gut microbiome and may inhibit growth of harmful bacteria. This supports optimal immune function and gut barrier integrity.

6. **POSSIBLE TREATMENT FOR INFLAMMATION:** Preliminary research shows hydrogen may improve inflammatory conditions like rheumatoid arthritis. More studies are still needed in this area but results are promising.

7. **BRAIN HEALTH:** Hydrogen protects neurons from oxidative stress and may help prevent age-related cognitive decline. It crosses the blood-brain barrier allowing benefits to reach the brain.

4. SUFFICIENT SLEEP:

Prioritizing quality sleep is crucial for overall health and well-being. I aim to get 7-8 hours of sleep each night, allowing my body to rest, recover, and rejuvenate. A good night's sleep enhances cognitive function, strengthens the immune system, and improves mood and emotional resilience.

5. STRESS MANAGEMENT:

In our hectic lives, stress can take a toll on our health. To combat this, I incorporate stress management techniques into my routine. This includes practicing mindfulness, deep breathing exercises, and engaging in activities I enjoy, such as reading, listening to music, or spending time in nature. Taking regular breaks and setting realistic goals also help me maintain a healthy work-life balance.

6. REGULAR HEALTH CHECK-UPS:

Prevention is better than cure, so I make it a habit to schedule regular health check-ups. These visits allow me to monitor my overall health, detect any potential issues early on, and seek appropriate medical advice if needed.

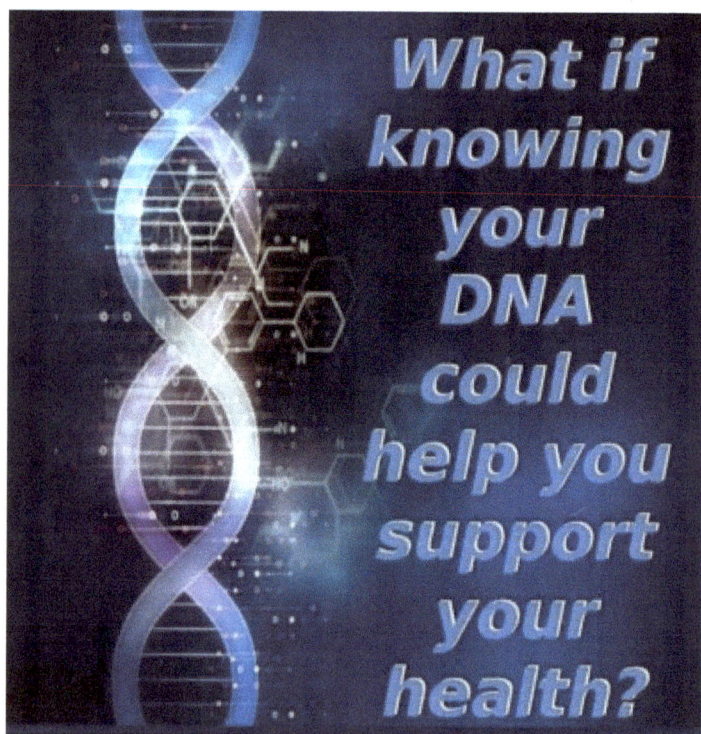

CHAPTER 2

What if knowing your DNA could help you support your health?

WHAT IF KNOWING YOUR DNA COULD REALLY HELP SUPPORT YOUR HEALTH?

When you focus on the importance of nutrition and lifestyle habits, you learn about the "macronutrients" (protein, carbohydrates, and fats) and the role they play in keeping your body functioning as it should. It is important to discuss micronutrients such as Vitamin D, Zinc, Magnesium, etc. and the importance of getting them in your diet. Creating that balanced diet that works for you based on what your genetics reveal about your needs is key to optimal health.

But what if there was even more information you could gain from your DNA? What if knowing your genetic makeup could provide personalized insights into how to take care of your body and prevent potential health issues? This is where the concept of genetic testing comes in. By analyzing your DNA, genetic testing can identify any variations or mutations that may impact your health. These variations can range from traits such as eye color to more serious conditions like a predisposition to certain diseases.

With this knowledge, you can work with healthcare professionals to develop a personalized plan that takes into account your genetic makeup, lifestyle habits, and nutrition needs. This approach goes beyond just general recommendations for a healthy lifestyle and instead focuses on what specifically works best for you.

As I mentioned, in 2019 my body started shutting down. I lost 30 pounds in 6 months, my muscle tone disappeared, my legs started to look like my arms and I was losing my strength and vitality. I went to 3 different doctors, including a Blood & Cancer specialist who did not find what was wrong. This is the point where a friend of mine, who was becoming well versed in epigenetic testing, suggested I let her test me to see if there was a genetic problem. I agreed and waited patiently for the results.

When the results came back, she did a quick review and recommended I go see the holistic doctor she was working with. So I scheduled and planned the trip to Austin, TX. It was the results of this testing and the interface with a Neurobiologist, Neuro-Immune & Genetic Specialist that started to turn my world around and start healing..

Meanwhile, I had scheduled an appointment with another holistic doctor who is a kinesiologist/chiropractor with his own line of nutritional supplements. He found another problem....a parasite running rampant throughout my body, in every organ. Yes, my body was shutting down quickly. I needed to detox and a parasite treatment ASAP.

The testing also showed that some of my health issues were caused by my genetic makeup, rather than just environmental factors. This knowledge helped me to understand my body and its limitations better, and allowed me to make more informed decisions about my health.

The kinesiologist found a clinical doctor who was five miles from my home. Great news! I made the needed appointment for a consultation. After initial testing, I was put on a strict protocol and parasite detox which would last for the next four months.

I followed the protocols as instructed. After two months I already started to feel better, and after four months I had a renewed sense of energy. My skin was healthier, my brain felt more alert and I had less cravings for sugar.

Today, I am grateful to say that I have regained most of my health and vitality. I still see the holistic doctors regularly to monitor my progress and make any necessary adjustments. But most importantly, I have learned the importance of taking care of myself holistically – addressing not only physical symptoms but also considering emotional, mental, and spiritual factors.

Through this experience, I have become an advocate for holistic health and wellness. I have shared my story with many others and have encouraged them to consider a holistic approach to their own health concerns. I believe that our bodies are complex systems, and addressing all aspects of our well-being is crucial for achieving true healing and lasting vitality.

I now realize that my initial skepticism about holistic medicine was misguided. While traditional medical treatments certainly have their place, incorporating holistic practices like nutrition, exercise, stress management, and self-care can greatly enhance our overall health and well-being.

So if you're struggling with any health issues or simply want to improve your overall wellness, I highly recommend considering a holistic approach. Consult with a trusted holistic practitioner or do some research on your own to find out what methods may work best for you. Remember, our bodies are unique and what works for one person may not necessarily work for another.

One of the key principles of holistic medicine is treating the root cause of an issue rather than just its symptoms. This means looking at the bigger picture and addressing underlying issues that may be contributing to your health problems. For example, instead of just prescribing medication for headaches, a holistic practitioner might also explore potential dietary triggers or stressors that could be causing them.

In addition to addressing physical ailments, holistic medicine also recognizes the connection between mind, body, and spirit. This means taking care of our mental and emotional well-being is just as important as our physical health. Techniques such as meditation, yoga, and mindfulness can help us manage stress and improve our overall well-being.

Holistic medicine places a strong emphasis on prevention. Instead of waiting for symptoms to arise and treating them reactively, holistic practitioners focus on promoting healthy lifestyle choices to prevent illness from occurring in the first place. This can include recommendations for proper nutrition, exercise, and stress management techniques.

Another key aspect of holistic medicine is individualized treatment. Rather than using a one-size-fits-all approach, holistic practitioners take into consideration each person's unique needs and circumstances when creating a treatment plan. This personalized approach allows for more effective and tailored care that addresses the root cause of an issue rather than just its symptoms. Our DNA is unique and so are our bodies, which is why it makes sense to approach healthcare in a personalized way.

In conclusion, holistic medicine offers a comprehensive approach to health and wellness by addressing not only physical ailments but also mental, emotional, and spiritual well-being. With its focus on prevention, patient empowerment, and individualized treatment, it offers a more holistic and sustainable approach to healthcare. Incorporating healthy lifestyle habits such as proper nutrition, regular exercise, and stress management techniques can also greatly contribute to overall health and well-being. By combining both traditional medical practices with holistic approaches, we can achieve optimal health for our mind, body, and soul. Remember, true health is not just the absence of disease but rather a state of complete physical, mental, emotional, and spiritual balance.

As I continue on my journey, I am so grateful for the knowledge and tools that kinesiology has provided me with. It has been life-changing! I have a newfound appreciation of how amazing our bodies are and what we can accomplish when we work together in harmony. Thank you kinesiology!

But what exactly did the testing show the genetic doctor? I was totally confused looking at the results as this was all a totally new language that I had to become very familiar with. The more I learned, the more passionate I became. Read on to learn why.

EAT well FEEL good

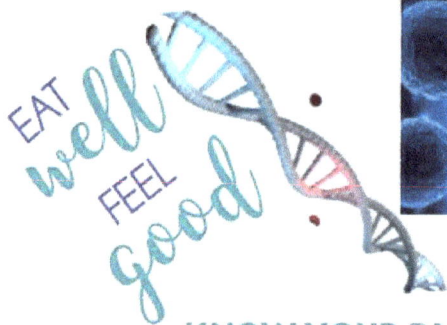

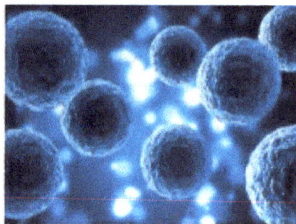

KNOW YOUR DNA,
KNOW YOUR HEALTH
with
YourDailyNourishment

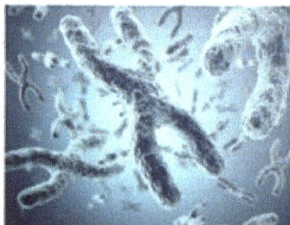

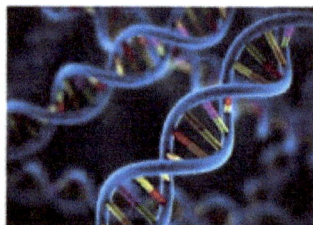

CHAPTER 3

UNDERSTANDING YOUR GENETIC CODE

The first step in understanding your genetic code is to learn the language it speaks. The most commonly used language is called "DNA" or Deoxyribonucleic Acid. This complex molecule contains all the information necessary for life, including instructions on how a person should look, function and develop over time. By studying this molecule, scientists are able to learn about individuals' genetic make-up and traits.

The next step is to gather the necessary data from a person's DNA. This can be done through various methods such as sequencing the entire genome or using targeted gene panels that look at specific genes associated with a particular condition or trait.

After the analysis has been completed, scientists can begin to interpret the results. This involves looking at all of the variants that have been identified and assessing their potential impact on a person's health.

Modern genetics has revolutionized the way in which we understand the human body and our predisposition to certain diseases. By examining a person's genetic code, researchers have unlocked the secrets of how our genes influence our health and wellbeing. This knowledge has been used to develop treatments and therapies that are tailored specifically for each person, offering them increased chances of success in managing their condition or disease, identifying potential risk factors for certain conditions, and enabling us to take preventative measures and reduce our chances of developing serious illnesses.

The potential applications of modern genetics are vast, ranging from diagnostics to therapeutics. For example, genetic testing can be used for early detection of cancer or other diseases. Genetic tests can be used to identify potential drug targets for treating various diseases, such as cancer or Alzheimer's disease.

Furthermore, gene therapy is an emerging field in which genes are modified to treat certain conditions, like muscular dystrophy or cystic fibrosis. Advances in genetic engineering could lead to the development of new treatments for currently incurable diseases such as HIV/AIDS.

Modern genetics has tremendous potential to improve healthcare and reduce suffering from life-threatening illnesses. By understanding the role of genetics in health and disease, scientists can develop innovative treatments for a wide range of conditions. This could have significant implications for improving both quality of life and longevity.

I have become a firm believer in the science of epigenetics and nutritional genomics because of where my health was four years ago to where it is today.

Understanding Your Genetic Code

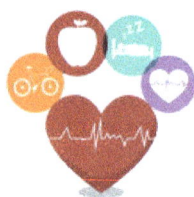

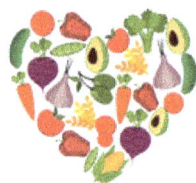

YourDailyNourishment

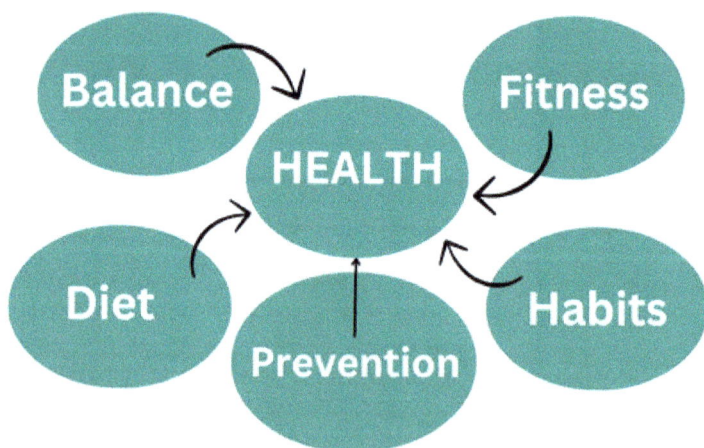

Balance

Fitness

HEALTH

Diet

Prevention

Habits

CHAPTER 4

WHAT CAN DNA TELL ME ABOUT MY HEALTH?

Epigenetics is the study of changes in gene expression or cellular phenotype that do not involve alterations to the underlying DNA sequence. It can provide insights into how your genes interact with your environment, lifestyle, and experiences. Here are some ways epigenetics can inform you about your health:

- **DISEASE RISK:** Epigenetic changes can influence your susceptibility to certain diseases. For example, changes in DNA methylation patterns may be associated with an increased or decreased risk of developing conditions like cancer, diabetes, or cardiovascular diseases.

- **ENVIRONMENTAL IMPACT:** Epigenetics reveals how your lifestyle and environment can affect gene expression. Factors such as diet, stress, exposure to toxins, and physical activity can leave epigenetic marks on your DNA, influencing health outcomes.

- **AGING:** Epigenetic modifications play a role in the aging process. Studying these changes can provide insights into how and why cells age, potentially leading to interventions for age-related conditions.

- **RESPONSE TO THERAPIES:** Epigenetic information can be used to predict how an individual might respond to certain treatments. This personalized approach, known as pharmacogenomics, aims to optimize drug efficacy and minimize side effects based on an individual's genetic and epigenetic profile.

- **INHERITED TRAITS:** Epigenetic modifications can be passed down from one generation to the next. Understanding these inherited epigenetic patterns may shed light on the transmission of certain traits and conditions within families.

- **DRUG DEVELOPMENT:** Epigenetics has also played a critical role in drug development. By identifying specific genetic and epigenetic markers associated with certain diseases or conditions, researchers are able to develop more targeted treatments that have higher rates of efficacy and fewer side effects. This personalized approach to medicine is known as pharmacogenomics and is revolutionizing the way we treat diseases.

- **PREVENTATIVE MEDICINE:** By understanding how our environment and lifestyle choices can impact our epigenetics, we are able to make more informed decisions about our health. This has led to the rise of preventative medicine, which aims to reduce the risk of developing certain diseases by promoting healthy behaviors and avoiding harmful environmental exposures.

- **PERSONALIZED HEALTHCARE:** The combination of genetic and epigenetic information allows for personalized healthcare plans tailored to an individual's unique needs. This can include screening for specific genetic mutations that may increase the risk of certain diseases, as well as tailoring treatments based on an individual's genetic makeup and epigenetic markers.

- **DISEASE DETECTION AND TREATMENT:** The ability to analyze a person's genome and epigenome has also greatly improved our ability to detect and treat diseases. With more targeted approaches, we are able to diagnose diseases earlier and develop more effective treatments that target the root cause rather than just managing symptoms.

- **ETHICAL CONSIDERATIONS:** While these advancements in understanding genetics and epigenetics have greatly benefited the field of medicine, they also raise ethical considerations. There is a concern about genetic discrimination, where individuals may face discrimination based on their genetic information or predisposition to certain diseases.

In simpler terms:

Imagine your body is like a book, and your genes are the words written in it. Epigenetics is like the highlighting, underlining, and notes made in the margins that don't change the words but tell you how to read and understand them.

Remember, while the book's notes are helpful, they're not the whole story. Other things like your choices and surroundings also matter. If you're curious about your book, it's a good idea to talk to a doctor or someone who understands these things to get the full picture of your health story.

Once I realized that our genes could affect how our bodies take in and use nutrients, I got really curious. How do our genetic tendencies influence our energy levels, sleep patterns, digestion, and the way we age? Everyone aims to age in a healthy way. Your unique DNA report can provide you with a clear understanding of what your body specifically requires and the reasons behind it.

There are so many good things that the results of your DNA Health Tests can alert you to. I will go deeper into this in the next chapters. But I will highlight a few here for now.

Let's start with sleep and the importance of sleep on our bodies.

Sleep impacts your mental clarity, emotional regulation, mood, and overall physical health. Did you know that our genetics can play a role in how well we sleep and how much we need? Some of us may be more genetically predisposed to being night owls, while others are early birds. Certain genetic variations can also affect our quality of sleep and risk for certain sleep disorders. Our genes can also play a role in determining our sleep patterns. Some people may have certain genetic variations that make them more prone to sleep disorders such as insomnia or sleep apnea. By being aware of these potential risks, you can take steps to improve your sleep hygiene and seek professional help if necessary. By understanding your genetic profile, you can make lifestyle changes to optimize your sleep habits and improve your overall health

How about *digestion*? Our genes influence how we metabolize food, absorb nutrients, and even react to certain foods. For example, some people may have a genetic variation that makes them more sensitive to gluten or lactose intolerance.

Knowing this information can help you tailor your diet to better suit your body's needs and avoid potential digestive issues.

Digestive issues such as irritable bowel syndrome (IBS) and Crohn's disease can also have a genetic component. By understanding your genetic predispositions, you can work with your doctor to manage these conditions and potentially prevent them from developing in the first place. Our gut health is also linked to our mental health, with studies showing a connection between gut bacteria and conditions like anxiety and depression.

How do your gene expressions link to mental health, anxiety and depression?

Research has shown that our gut microbiome, the community of microorganisms in our digestive tract, plays a crucial role in our overall health and well-being. These microorganisms help to break down food, produce essential nutrients, and support our immune system. When there is an imbalance or disruption in the gut microbiome, it can have a ripple effect on other systems in the body, including our mental health.

Just as certain genetic variations can impact how our bodies respond to *stress and inflammation.* This can make individuals more susceptible to conditions like anxiety and depression. For example, studies have found a link between certain variations in serotonin-related genes and an increased risk of developing depression.

The BDNF gene, which plays a role in the growth and survival of neurons in the brain, has also been linked to mental health. Variations in this gene have been associated with conditions like schizophrenia and bipolar disorder. The coffeeberry extract found in "RED" coffee has been shown to increase the production of BDNF, potentially providing support for those who may have genetic variations in this gene.

But genetics are not the only factor at play when it comes to mental health. Environmental factors, such as our diet and lifestyle choices, also have a significant impact. For example, a diet high in processed foods and sugar has been linked to an increased risk of depression and other mental health disorders.

That's why we've formulated our products with ingredients that not only provide essential nutrients for overall well-being but also specifically target gut health. By promoting a healthy balance of gut bacteria, we can support proper digestion and absorption of nutrients, which is crucial for brain function.

In addition to nourishing your body with essential vitamins and minerals, there are products that also contain adaptogenic herbs that help your body cope with stress. Chronic stress can have a detrimental effect on mental health, leading to anxiety and mood disorders. By incorporating adaptogens into your daily routine, you can better manage stress and support your mental well-being.

I understand that taking care of your mental health is just as important as taking care of your physical health. That's why I chose a company which created a line of products that not only prioritize nutrition but also aim to improve overall mood and cognitive function. The goal is to empower you to take control of your mental health journey through natural and effective means.

So whether you're dealing with a specific mental health condition or simply looking for ways to improve your overall well-being, their adaptogen-based products can offer the support and balance your mind and body need. Let's explore how adaptogens work and how they can benefit your mental health specifically.

What exactly are adaptogens? These are non-toxic plants that have been used for centuries in traditional medicine practices to help the body adapt to stressors. They work by regulating the body's stress response and promoting a sense of calm and balance. This is achieved through their ability to modulate hormones such as cortisol, which is often referred to as the "stress hormone."

By reducing cortisol levels, adaptogens can help alleviate symptoms of anxiety and depression, which are often linked to high levels of this hormone. But it's not just about lowering cortisol; these powerful plants also have the ability to regulate other hormones and neurotransmitters, such as serotonin and dopamine, which play a crucial role in our mood and overall mental well-being.

One of the most well-known adaptogens is ashwagandha, often referred to as "Indian ginseng." Studies have shown that this herb can decrease cortisol levels by up to 30% while also improving symptoms of anxiety and depression.

Another popular adaptogen is rhodiola rosea, commonly found in arctic regions. This plant has been used for centuries in traditional medicine to combat fatigue and increase focus. It works by increasing the production of serotonin and dopamine, helping to boost mood and cognitive function.

Ginseng is another widely used adaptogen that has been shown to improve the body's resistance to stress and fatigue. It also has anti-inflammatory properties, making it beneficial for those with chronic pain or inflammation.

Holy basil, also known as tulsi, is a lesser-known but powerful adaptogen that has been used in Ayurvedic medicine for centuries. It has been shown to have anti-anxiety and antidepressant effects by regulating cortisol levels and promoting relaxation.

Reishi mushrooms have gained popularity in recent years for their adaptogenic properties. These fungi have been used in traditional Chinese medicine for thousands of years and are believed to enhance immune function, reduce stress, and improve overall well-being.

While each adaptogen may have different mechanisms of action, they all work towards the common goal of helping our bodies adapt to stressors and maintain homeostasis. This makes them a valuable addition to any wellness routine, especially for those dealing with chronic stress or health issues.

Now that you have an understanding of what adaptogens are and their potential benefits, it's important to note that not all adaptogens are created equal. It's crucial to do your research and consult with a healthcare professional before incorporating them into your regimen. Additionally, be cautious of products claiming to contain adaptogens but may actually just be using the term as a marketing ploy.

Adaptogens offer a natural and holistic approach to managing stress and improving overall well-being. With various options available, there is an adaptogen out there for everyone. Just remember to always prioritize safety and consult with experts before adding them into your routine. Whether it's through supplements, teas, or even incorporating adaptogenic foods into your diet, these powerful herbs have the potential to transform your health and help you better manage stress in a sustainable way.

So next time you're feeling overwhelmed, instead of reaching for that second cup of coffee or sugary snack, consider giving adaptogens a try. With their ability to balance and restore the body, they may just be the missing piece in achieving optimal health and wellness. Take control of your stress levels today and explore the world of adaptogens – your mind and body will thank you!

Next, our gut microbiome also plays a key role in the production of neurotransmitters, such as serotonin and dopamine, which are essential for regulating mood and emotion. When there is an imbalance in the gut microbiome, it can impact the levels of these neurotransmitters and lead to symptoms of anxiety or depression.

This connection between the gut microbiome and mental health highlights the importance of maintaining a healthy balance in our gut bacteria. This includes eating a diverse and nutritious diet, managing stress through practices like meditation or exercise, and taking probiotic supplements if needed.

This has caused a problem with a drug that had been prescribed by a Neurologist for my depression. Sertraline, an SSRI drug, caused me to hallucinate. I was told, "it wasn't the drug." It wasn't until I had my testing and reading over my reports that I found that because of the SLC6A4 variant that I carry, I may have less than optimal response to SSRI drugs. So no more SSRI's for me.

It's also worth noting that our *environment* can greatly influence our gut microbiome. Factors such as exposure to toxins, antibiotics, and even socioeconomic status can all play a role in disrupting the delicate balance of our gut bacteria. This is why it's important to not only focus on dietary changes, but also addressing any external factors that may be contributing to gut imbalances.

In addition to genetics, environmental factors can also play a significant role in our mental health. Chronic stress, exposure to toxins, poor diet, and lack of exercise can all contribute to imbalances in the gut microbiome and trigger inflammation in the body.

On the other hand, taking care of our gut health by incorporating probiotic-rich foods like yogurt and fermented vegetables, as well as prebiotic foods like bananas and garlic, can help support a healthy balance of microorganisms in our digestive tract. Managing stress through techniques such as mindfulness meditation or yoga can also have a positive impact on our gut health.

Furthermore, changes in diet can greatly influence the diversity and abundance of bacteria in the gut. Switching to a whole foods-based diet that includes plenty of fruits, vegetables, and healthy fats can not only improve overall physical health but also promote a more diverse microbiome.

It's important to remember that every individual is unique, and what works for one person may not work for another. Consulting with a healthcare professional or registered dietician who specializes in gut health can be beneficial in creating a personalized plan for improving gut health. Having your DNA health results with you to help the doctors understand your blueprint can be a game changer for your health journey.

By addressing both internal and external factors, we can take control of our gut health and promote overall well-being. So the next time you sit down for a meal, remember that you are not just feeding yourself, but also your gut microbiome. Choose whole, unprocessed foods and incorporate probiotic-rich options like yogurt, kimchi, and kombucha into your diet. And don't forget to manage stress levels and get enough sleep to keep your gut happy.

Our gut is often referred to as our "second brain" due to its complex network of neurons that communicates with our central nervous system. Therefore, taking care of our gut can also have a positive impact on our mood, emotions, and overall mental well-being.

So let's make a conscious effort to prioritize our gut health by nourishing it with nutrient-dense foods and creating a healthy and balanced lifestyle. Not only will it improve our digestion, but also benefit our overall health and happiness. Let's give our gut the love and attention it deserves!

When choosing a probiotic, the 3 Essential Probiotic Cultures for a Healthy Gut are as follows.

BACILLUS SUBTILIS

- Naturally occurring in soil and compost.
- Resilient spore-forming bacteria surviving extreme conditions.
- Remains dormant in the digestive tract, activating in the colon.
- Supports bowel regularity and safeguards the gut-blood barrier.
- Promotes a healthy balance of good to bad bacteria in the gut.

BACILLUS COAGULANS

- Found in fermented foods like sauerkraut and kimchi.
- Forms endospores for survival in the gastric tract.

- Offers comprehensive probiotic support in smaller doses.
- Reduces gas, bloating, and abdominal discomfort.
- Enhances bowel regularity.

BACILLUS CLAUSII

- Spore-forming probiotic with a safe profile.
- Naturally present in plant soil and fresh-grown vegetables.
- Survives and replicates after exposure to gastric fluids.
- Resistant to acidity, thriving in the gastrointestinal tract.
- Strengthens the colon lining, fights harmful microbes, and protects against digestive issues.

Genetics also play a role in the production of neurotransmitters, which are responsible for regulating mood and emotions. However, our gut bacteria also have the ability to produce these neurotransmitters, making their health just as important in managing stress and promoting mental well-being.

But probiotics aren't just beneficial for our physical and mental health, they can also improve our skin's appearance. The gut-skin axis is a complex relationship between our gut microbiome and the health of our skin. Studies have shown that certain probiotic strains, such as Lactobacillus rhamnosus and Bifidobacterium bifidum, can help alleviate symptoms of inflammatory skin conditions like acne and eczema.

Another surprising benefit of probiotics is their potential role in weight management.

PLEASE DO YOUR RESEARCH BEFORE BUYING A PRE/PRO/POST BIOTIC to ensure it does not have fillers and that is it clean.

In addition to diet and digestion, Our genes also influence our overall physical health and predisposition to certain diseases. For example, a genetic test can determine if you have an increased risk for conditions like heart disease, diabetes, or cancer. With this knowledge, you can make lifestyle changes and work with your doctor on preventative measures to minimize your risk and promote better health.

Knowing this information can help individuals better understand their risk for certain disorders and seek appropriate treatments or preventative measures. It can also help break stigmas surrounding mental health by showing that it is not solely based on personal choices or character flaws.

And what about *exercise*? Our genes also play a role in our athletic abilities and recovery time. Certain genetic variations can affect our muscle composition, metabolism, and injury risk. Why does DNA affect our athletic abilities? It all comes back to the individual variations in our genetic code that make us unique. By understanding your genetic makeup, you can personalize your workout routine to maximize results and prevent potential injuries.

But genetics is not the only factor that contributes to our health and well-being. Our environment, lifestyle choices, and access to healthcare also play a significant role. By understanding our genetic predispositions, we can take steps towards creating a personalized approach to living a healthier life.

If you have a family history of heart disease and discover through genetic testing that you carry certain risk factors, you can work with your doctor to closely monitor your heart health and make necessary changes to your diet and exercise routine. This proactive approach can help reduce your chances of developing heart disease.

Genetic testing also has implications for reproductive health. For couples planning on starting a family, knowing their carrier status for genetic disorders can help them make informed decisions about family planning and preventative measures. This information can also be valuable for those undergoing fertility treatments, as it may impact the success rate.

Aside from health-related benefits, genetic testing can also provide insight into our ancestry and origins. Through DNA analysis, we can discover our unique ethnic background and even connect with long-lost relatives. This can be a meaningful experience for individuals looking to learn more about their identity and heritage.

However, it's important to note that genetic testing is not a crystal ball. It cannot predict future health outcomes with 100% accuracy. It's also crucial to have proper guidance and counseling before and after taking a genetic test. Genetic counselors are trained professionals who can help individuals navigate the complexities of genetic testing and understand their results.

So why choose one over the other? The truth is that both epigenetics and nutritional genomics are vital components in unlocking the secrets of optimal health. They complement each other in providing a holistic view of how our bodies function at a molecular level. Unlike genetic changes, *epigenetic changes are reversible* and do not change your DNA sequence, but they can change how your body reads a DNA sequence.

In summary, genetic testing can be a valuable tool for individuals to gain insight into their health and ancestry. With proper education and guidance, it can empower us to make informed decisions about our well-being and give us a deeper understanding of ourselves. So whether you're considering genetic testing for health reasons or out of curiosity, it's essential to do your research and consult with healthcare professionals before making any decisions. Remember, knowledge is power, but it's how we use that knowledge that truly matters.

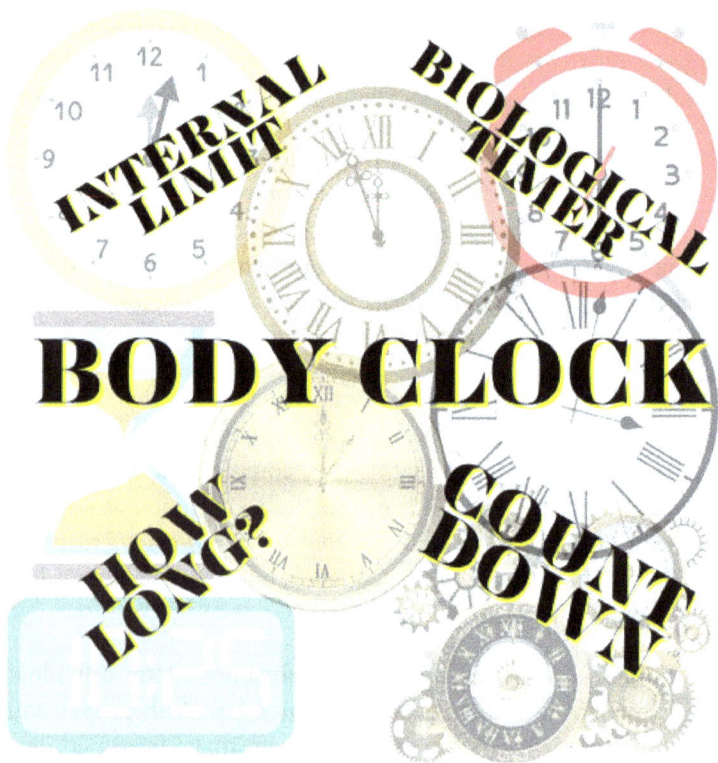

INTERNAL LIMIT

BIOLOGICAL TIMER

BODY CLOCK

HOW LONG?

COUNT DOWN

CHAPTER 5

CLOSING THE GAP

Closing the gap of your lifespan: healthy eating

J ust to be clear, genetic testing analyzes your DNA to reveal variations in your genes that may cause illness or disease. Nutrigenomic testing is a specific genetic test showing an individual's unique nutritional needs.

With the help of nutritional genomics testing, you can learn about your unique nutritional needs and make informed dietary changes to support your health and longevity. By understanding which food groups provide essential nutrients with beneficial biochemicals for your body's individual needs, you can personalize a diet plan that maximizes its potential benefits.

In addition to uncovering genetic–based nutritional insights, you can also explore how food affects your wellbeing. For example, it can provide clues on how particular foods may trigger a *positive or negative response* in your body. In this way, it gives you the opportunity to become an active participant in optimizing your lifestyle for health and wellness. These are functions of the on/off switches that are activated or deactivated.

Genetic expression is all about how our genetic information gets translated into instructions for creating proteins or other molecules. It's like flipping a switch to turn on a gene, and in more scientific terms, it's called gene expression. Our genes use a process called methylation to fix our DNA and control whether genes are active or inactive.

When DNA is damaged, it doesn't send messages to the rest of the body properly. In cells that don't replicate, this can lead to accelerated aging. Our lifestyle choices, like the food we eat, the chemicals we expose ourselves to, and the environment we live in, can either increase or decrease stress on our DNA, affecting gene expression. Taking care of our DNA is crucial!

Additionally, understanding our gene expression through nutrigenomics can also help us make targeted dietary changes to support specific health concerns. For instance, someone with a family history of heart disease may be able to reduce their risk by incorporating more foods that support heart health into their diet.

So let's start with food. It is well known that the body needs certain nutrients to function properly. The DNA Nutritional Genomics Test can give information on what food would be beneficial for you and which one might not be a good option.

For example, if you test positive for a gene variant associated with celiac disease, then it could indicate you should avoid gluten-containing foods to reduce potential symptoms. Additionally, the test can also provide insight into how you might react to certain medications. It could suggest if a drug would be more or less effective or cause an adverse reaction. This could help you make better decisions about treatments and dosages with your physician.

These tests can also be used to understand how your body metabolizes certain foods or pills, helping you to make the best health and nutrition decisions. With all of this information at your fingertips, it's easier than ever to take control of your own health.

The benefits of nutritional genomics aren't limited to giving individuals an understanding of their own health risks. With the rise in genetic testing technology, more companies are beginning to offer personalized recommendations based on an individual's genetic makeup. This can be incredibly useful when it comes to making decisions about which vitamins and supplements are best for your body, or even which foods you should add to your diet. By taking into account an individual's unique DNA profile, companies can provide tailored advice and recommendations that can help improve overall health and wellness.

Overall, the benefits of DNA testing are vast and can help individuals gain valuable insights into their ancestry, health, and lifestyle. From finding long lost relatives to discovering new ways to improve your personal wellbeing, the possibilities of what you can uncover are truly endless. With its ever-growing popularity, DNA testing promises a fascinating journey of self-discovery that will continue to evolve as technology advances. Here is how nutritional genomics works!

WHAT IS AN ACTIONABLE SNP?

An actionable single nucleotide polymorphism (SNP) is a variant in the sequence of your DNA that can be used to determine how certain nutrients or food compounds may affect you. This information can help you choose foods to include (or avoid) in your diet that will best support your health goals and needs. For example, an actionable SNP could reveal if you have a genetic predisposition towards developing diabetes. Knowing this could help you make dietary and lifestyle changes to reduce your risk of disease. Understanding how certain foods may interact with your body can also aid in medication decisions, as some medications are metabo-lized differently by individuals with specific SNPs.

Actionable SNP testing is only one way to gain insight into your nutrition needs. Working with a qualified healthcare provider or registered dietitian or test provider can also provide invaluable knowledge about personalized nutrition recommendations based on your individual goals and medical history. They can assess your current diet and lifestyle habits to determine if there are any areas for improvement. They can also provide guidance on tailored sup-plementation based on your individual nutrient needs. Ultimately, this can help you achieve improved health outcomes through ev-idence-based nutritional decisions. But, without knowing what your body does with the nutrition won't give you the right answer or the most effective solution. This is where DNA testing can come in.

Taking these steps towards personalizing your nutrition is an im-portant part of staying healthy and achieving long-term health goals. By empowering yourself with knowledge, you can take con-trol of your health journey and make informed decisions about how to live a healthier life.

One of the most practical ways to personalize nutrition is to track what you eat. This allows you to be mindful of your food choices and monitor your nutrient intake. As you become more aware of what you are eating, you may realize that your diet is lacking in certain nutrients or that there are certain foods that don't work well with your body. With this information, you can then make changes to better meet your individual needs.

Different bodies respond differently to different kinds of foods, so it's important to find out what works best for you. This could in-volve keeping a food journal or experimenting with new recipes and ingredients.

Here is an analogy for you.

Just as putting the wrong fuel in your vehicle disrupts its smooth operation, our bodies function optimally when fueled correctly. Imagine pouring regular gas into a diesel engine or vice versa – the result? Inefficiency, a lack of smooth performance, and potential long-term damage. The parallel is striking: the foods we choose significantly impact our body's efficiency and overall well-being. Choose your body's fuel wisely for a smoother and more impactful journey through life.

To find out which foods work best for you, pay attention to how your body responds after eating certain meals. Do you feel energized? Do you notice any bloating or discomfort? Does your nose start to run? Does your throat get scratchy? This can also vary based on factors like age, metabolism, and activity level. There are more than likely food sensitivity issues.

Another aspect of personalizing nutrition is understanding portion sizes. While there are general guidelines for serving sizes, everyone's caloric needs are different. A petite person may require less food than someone who is taller and more physically active. Learning what amount of food makes your body feel good (not too full or overly hungry) can greatly enhance your overall well-being.

Overall, personalizing nutrition means finding ways to better meet your individual needs and preferences when it comes to food. This could involve tracking what you eat, experimenting with different foods and recipes, and working with a dietician or other health professional. With the right plan in place, you can enjoy a more nutritious and balanced diet that fits your lifestyle. Work with a health professional or dietician who can help you develop an individualized eating plan based on your specific needs. *Please make sure they know your DNA blueprint.*

They say, **MINDSET IS EVERYTHING!**

The key is to be patient with yourself when creating or altering your nutrition plan. You may need to try out different approaches before finally finding something that works for you. Remember that everyone has unique needs and preferences, so it's important to find what works best for you. Varying your diet and eating a variety of nutrient-dense foods can help to ensure that you are getting all the necessary vitamins and minerals for optimal health. Make sure to pay attention to any food allergies or sensitivities that you might have.

By taking the time to plan and prepare your meals, you can look forward to a healthier lifestyle and long-term positive effects on your wellbeing. It's important to consult with a doctor or registered dietician if you have any questions or concerns about your nutrition plan.

What I have learned is if your sinuses become inflamed or your nose starts to run after eating certain foods, then it is best to avoid them and look for alternatives. You may just have a food sensitivity due to a gene mutation. I have seen people change their diet, and it has made a huge difference in how they felt afterwards. It is great to listen to your body when you are planning out your meals.*

Additionally, tracking your intake can help you identify which foods may be causing inflammation or other undesired reactions in the body. Also, keep an eye on portion sizes when eating—too much of even a healthy food can still lead to weight gain.

Physical activity is just as important as diet when it comes to overall health. Regular exercise can help regulate hormones, improve digestion, and reduce stress. It's important to choose an activity that you enjoy and to stick with it as part of a healthy lifestyle.

No matter what your diet looks like or how much exercise you get, it is important to care for yourself in all aspects: physically, emotionally, and mentally. Consider talking to a healthcare professional if you have any further questions or concerns. It's never too late to start taking steps towards a healthier you!

*Please note that this article is for informational purposes only and should not be taken as medical advice. Please consult a doctor or medical professional if you have any questions or concerns about your health & wellness.

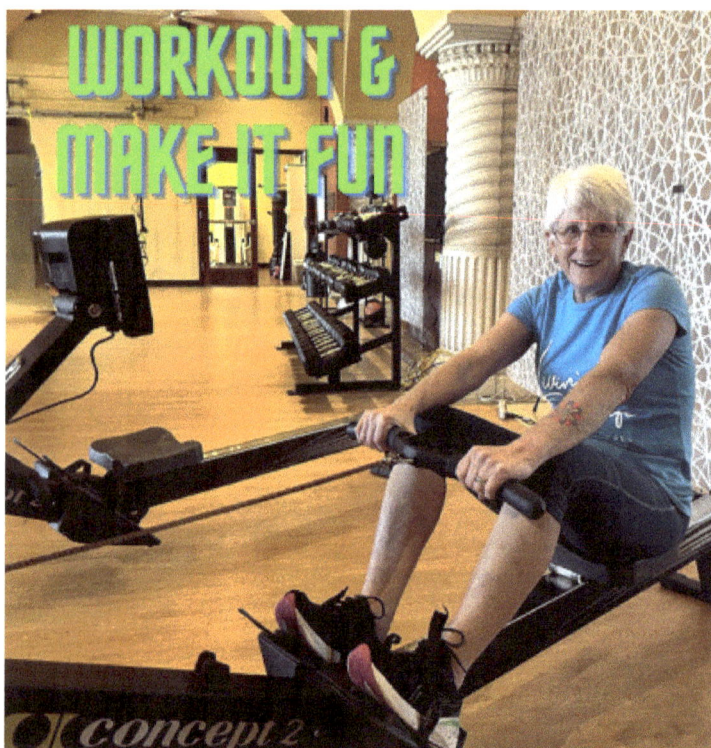

WORKOUT &
MAKE IT FUN

CHAPTER 6

GETTING PHYSICAL: STAYING ACTIVE

A s well as eating right, taking part in regular physical activity is essential for good health. Regular physical activity has been shown to help reduce the risk of many chronic diseases and can help improve your overall well being. Consider talking to a healthcare professional before beginning any new exercise program so that you can find something that's best suited for you.

Physical activity doesn't need to be boring; try to make it fun and enjoyable. Consider joining a sports team or taking part in an exercise class at the gym, or even look into activities like dance classes, swimming and yoga. Here in Florida, we play bocce, bike, walk, swim, water aerobics, zumba, yoga, pool volleyball, golf, bowling; the options are endless.

Take advantage of your gyms, YMCA, or other athletic center. Join a class for comradery and support. It is more fun when you have work out partners!

Remember that just 30 minutes of moderate-intensity physical activity every day can help improve your mental and physical health! Caring for your body goes beyond just diet and exercise. Make sure you get enough sleep, take breaks when needed, practice stress relief techniques like mindfulness or yoga, and seek social support from friends and family. All of these things make up an integral part of self-care that are often overlooked. Even using light weights, 2, 3, 5 pounds and doing movements with them watching a show will help your metabolism.

Don't forget to stay hydrated! Drinking water is essential for maintaining a healthy body and mind. It helps flush out toxins, regulates body temperature, and keeps your skin looking radiant. Make sure to carry a water bottle with you throughout the day and aim for at least 8 glasses of water per day.

Eating well is also crucial for overall health and fitness. Aim for a balanced diet that includes plenty of fruits, vegetables, whole grains, lean proteins, and healthy fats. Avoid processed foods and sugars as much as possible. Remember that fueling your body with nutritious food will give you the energy you need to conquer each day.

In addition to physical health, it's important to take care of your mental health as well.

Find something that you enjoy and make it a part of your routine, whether it's taking a walk in the park or playing sports with friends. It's important to prioritize your health…it is very important for overall wellbeing and happiness.

If possible, find activities that get you outdoors. Fresh air and natural sunlight can do wonders for clearing the mind and boosting your mood. Not only will regular physical activity make you feel better, but it can also help lower risk of chronic diseases such as heart disease or stroke in the long run. So don't forget to fit some exercise into your day!

Keeping up with regular check-ups and health screenings are also important for staying healthy. Make sure to schedule appointments when needed, or listen to your body if it's telling you something isn't feeling right. Staying on top of any potential health issues will help prevent serious problems down the line.

Most importantly, don't forget to take some time out of your day to relax. Taking some time for yourself can help relieve stress and give you an opportunity to just enjoy life without worrying about all the little things that may be stressing you out. So whether it's taking a nap, reading a book, or subscribing to a streaming service such as Netflix, find something that will give you a short break from the hustle and bustle of life.

Last but not least, don't forget to stay in touch with your friends and family. Keeping up relationships is important for both physical and mental health so make sure to carve out some time each week to catch up with those close to you!

These are just a few tips that can help you live a healthier lifestyle, but every individual is different so don't be afraid to experiment and find what works best for you. Remember, taking care of yourself is the key to being able to take on anything life throws at you!

Remember not to be discouraged if you don't reach your goals right away; health doesn't happen overnight! Have patience, and keep setting goals that you want to reach. Keep track of your progress and reward yourself with positive reinforcement when you do something right, it can help motivate you to continue making small changes towards a healthier you!

Good luck on your journey!

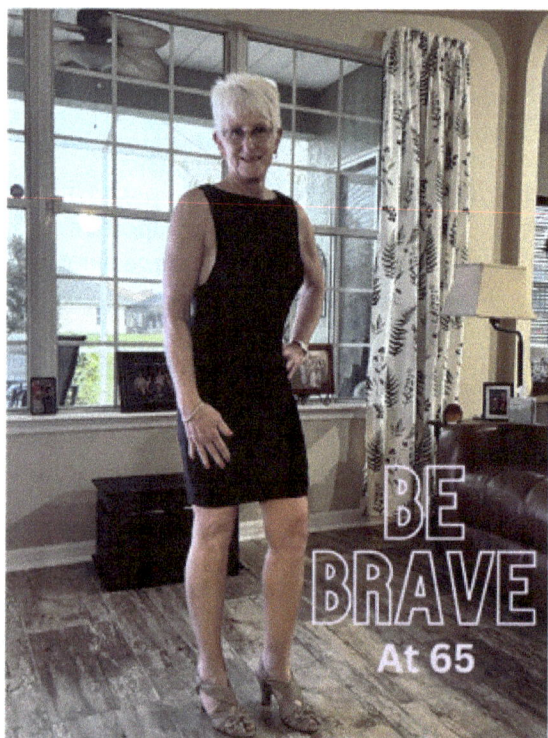

BE
BRAVE
At 65

CHAPTER 7

HEALTHSPAN VS BIOLOGICAL AGE

The goal of nutritional genomics is to support your healthspan and biological age through science-based analysis of your own genetic profile, and through nutritional supplementation in the right form and quantity specific to your DNA.

In this chapter, we'll explore ways that you can begin to uncover your unique genetic makeup and unlock the power of your genes. We'll also discuss strategies for managing your gene expression through diet, exercise, and lifestyle changes. Finally, we'll look at how genetic testing can help you discover your true biological age and design a personalized nutrition plan to optimize your gene expression for lifelong health. By understanding the power of epigenetics, you can transform your life by unlocking the secrets hidden within your genes. So let's dive in!

WHAT ABOUT THOSE CELLS?

Do you know what's behind them? It might be the best kept secret in the world of health and nutrition. Researchers are now discovering that our gene expression can influence how well we manage certain foods and respond to exercise.

HOW IS YOUR BIOLOGICAL AGE DETERMINED?

Biological age refers to our well-being and performance in relation to our chronological age, influenced by epigenetic modifications, cellular function, and the pace of deterioration. It varies among individuals, as lifestyle habits can impact chemical changes in our DNA, telomeres, and cells. Our comprehension of mortality and the rate of unhealthy aging has evolved, emphasizing that it is not solely determined by a numerical age.

Epigenetics is an incredibly powerful tool that can help you understand your unique genetic makeup and develop a personalized health plan to optimize gene expression for lifelong health. With the right knowledge, you can begin to unlock the power of your genes and transform your life.

Ready to learn more? Let's get started!

Our DNA contains instructions for making proteins and other molecules that are essential for our bodies to function. But our genes don't always express themselves in the same way. By understanding how epigenetics works, you can start to unlock the secrets hidden within your genes and design a personalized nutrition plan that will optimize your health for life.

The epicenter of the epigenetic revolution is nutrition. Locations of millions of DNA 'switches' that dictate how, when, and where in the body different genes turn on and off have been identified.

In the absence of these crucial switches known as regulatory DNA, genes remain inactive. Scientists globally have concentrated their efforts on pinpointing regulatory DNA to unravel the intricacies of genome functioning. With the aid of a cutting-edge technology developed through support from the National Human Genome Research Institute's ENCODE (ENCyclopedia Of DNA Elements) project, University of Washington researchers have crafted comprehensive maps outlining the specific locations of regulatory DNA in numerous types of living cells. Additionally, they have compiled a dictionary elucidating the instructions encoded within regulatory DNA – essentially the genome's programming language.

Healthy eating habits can help you control gene expression and make sure your body is functioning optimally. Eating a balanced diet that includes plenty of fruits, vegetables, and lean proteins will provide the nutrients needed for good health. Additionally, avoiding processed foods, added sugars, and unhealthy fats can help reduce inflammation and support proper gene expression.

When you take your epigenetic or nutritional genomics test you'll learn about which foods and supplements activate your genes and which ones suppress them. You'll learn how to make healthy lifestyle decisions that will have a positive effect on your gene expression, allowing you to live a longer, healthier life.

You'll also discover the power of environmental factors, such as stress and toxins, and how they can affect your gene expression. You'll also explore some of the cutting-edge epigenetic therapies that have revolutionized modern medicine. With this knowledge, you can begin to take control of your health and develop a unique plan for optimal living.

By exploring the science behind epigenetics, you can make better decisions about how to fuel your body with the right nutrients to provide it with all of the essential elements it needs for maximum health. You'll also gain insight into how your environment and lifestyle choices can affect the expression of your genes.

You'll learn about specific dietary strategies that can help you reprogram your gene expression and take control of your wellbeing, as well as discovering how to identify which epigenetic therapies are right for you. You'll also have access to valuable resources such as recipes, nutrition tips, lifestyle advice, and more to help you make the most out of your journey. Start exploring today and take control of your health!

Integrating epigenetics with exercise, nutrition, and lifestyle modifications allows you to establish an optimal environment for your body's well-being. This approach enables you to pinpoint potential sources of stress affecting your health and make necessary adjustments. Moreover, you can leverage epigenetics to assess the effectiveness of specific dietary or exercise routines and adapt them as required. Monitoring how environmental factors influence your health empowers you to identify areas for improvement, ensuring that you provide your body with the necessary support. The potential outcomes are vast!

Embrace *personalized epigenetic testing and analysis* to move beyond generic advice. Gain unique insights tailored to your body, allowing you to discover what works best for you. Don't hesitate any longer; start using epigenetics today to bring about lasting changes in both your body and your life. It's like tuning in to your cells' communication, similar to listening to your gut instincts!

SPEAKING OF CELLS, WHAT ARE HEALTHY CELLS VS UNHEALTHY CELLS?

It all started to make more sense when I read my epigenetic report. "Healthy cells have a soft, permeable cell membrane and allow for a healthy balance called homeostasis. When functioning nutrients get inside and waste products get out. Your healthy cells work to fight pathogens and have a life cycle where new ones are formed and old ones die. This is all part of the healthy aging process and supports or even reduces your biological age.

In contrast, unhealthy cells have hard, rigid, less permeable cell membranes. Since they do not function efficiently, these cells reduce the nutrients delivered to the cell nucleus and keep waste inside. The result is decreased cellular energy, increased unhealthy aging, and more vulnerability to pathogens. They get the nickname zombie cells because they just don't die!

WHAT ARE TELOMERES?

It is a repeating DNA sequence at the end of each chromosome. Telomeres have been compared to plastic tips on shoelaces, as they protect our chromosomes from damage and improve their stability with age. Every time a cell divides, part of the telomere gets shorter until it eventually becomes too short to protect the chromosome. When this happens, DNA information begins to degrade and the cell can no longer function properly, leading to aging.

WHICH FACTOR IS THE MOST RELIABLE MEASURE OF BIOLOGICAL AGE?

Telomere length has long been studied as a marker of biological age, but there is growing interest in other predictors. When telomeres get too short, cells enter a state called senescence. In this state, cells lose the ability to divide or perform vital functions like repairing damage or responding to signals from the environment. Rather than dying, these senescent cells accumulate in various tissues throughout the body, triggering inflammation and potentially contributing to the development of diseases.

Scientists view telomeres as indicators of aging and health, serving as biomarkers for cellular aging. Measuring telomere length allows a deeper understanding of how our bodies age and why individuals age at different rates. Lifestyle factors like diet, exercise, stress, and smoking may influence telomere length, offering insight into how our choices affect health and lifespan. Ongoing research explores potential treatments to restore or extend telomeres, aiming to slow the aging process.

Shortening telomeres can result in DNA strand breaks, increasing the risk of genetic mutations and diseases like cancer. Researchers examine how telomere length impacts health, considering their use as diagnostic tools for diseases. Future applications may involve monitoring disease progression and informing treatment decisions based on changes in telomere length.

In the quest for healthier aging, scientists explore lifestyle modifications and treatments to extend telomeres. Maintaining healthy telomeres through a balanced diet, regular exercise, stress reduction, adequate sleep, and quitting smoking may positively impact overall health and lifespan. Telomeres could potentially become a standard marker for assessing health, predicting disease risk and the onset of chronic diseases like heart disease and cancer. It's important to note that while more research on telomeres and aging is needed, comprehending their role in health equips us with a tool for prevention and early disease detection. Weight loss and metabolism are also affected by telomere length, as individuals who maintain a healthy weight and have good metabolic health tend to have longer telomeres. Additionally, certain medications such as aspirin and statins have been shown to slow down telomere shortening, though more studies are needed to determine their effectiveness in extending lifespan.

One of the key factors in maintaining healthy telomeres is proper nutrition. Consuming a diet rich in fruits, vegetables, whole grains, and lean proteins can provide the necessary vitamins and minerals for cellular repair and growth. In particular, foods high in antioxidants like berries, leafy greens, and nuts may help protect against oxidative stress that can lead to telomere shortening.

We can look at one person's DNA test results and see that they have a greater propensity toward developing diabetes, or we can compare two people's gene expressions to discover which diet might work best for each.

By taking advantage of the advances in genomics, you can now tailor a nutrition plan that is specific to your individual genetic makeup. This means that you can enjoy the foods that are best for your body type and be sure to get the most benefit from any physical activity that you take on. With this knowledge, you can make more informed decisions about which vitamins or supplements you might need, and even which recipes are most likely to help reach your desired result.

The potential of personalized nutrition is just beginning to be realized, and as technology advances, more precise recommendations can be made. By utilizing the accumulated knowledge of a variety of disciplines, we can create diets that optimize our health for our own unique biology— something that was never possible before. With this new capability, you have the power when it comes to nutrition in your hands. So get ready to take on a journey of discovery and learn more about your own individual health needs.

No matter your health goals, personalized nutrition can provide the answers you need to make sure that your diet is giving you the best possible outcomes. So take control and start exploring just what this new revolution in nutrition has to offer! You may be surprised at the individualized level of care you can get when it comes to taking charge of your own health and nutrition.

It is important to remember that personalized nutrition does not replace professional medical advice or the use of traditional treatments. Always consult with a healthcare professional before starting any new health routine. With the help of an experienced healthcare provider and/or nutritionist, and your DNA report, you can create a comprehensive plan that will work for your specific needs.

Why personalized nutrition? It stands as a potent tool, offering an individualized approach to dietary choices. By utilizing your genetic data and considering lifestyle factors, you can craft a plan specifically tailored to your unique needs. By taking the time to evaluate both your genetic makeup and lifestyle, you can be confident that your nutrition plan is precisely designed to meet your specific requirements.

The advantages of personalized nutrition are diverse, ranging from overall health improvements to increased energy levels and enhanced performance in physical activities, including sports. With personalized nutrition, you gain the ability to make informed decisions about your diet—what you eat and how much you consume—ensuring that your body receives the necessary nutrients to reach its full potential. This approach can contribute to maintaining a healthy healthspan and potentially slowing down biological aging.

Collaborating with an experienced healthcare professional can provide valuable insights into how your genes influence your body. Their guidance can be instrumental in creating a personalized nutrition plan that aligns with your unique genetic and lifestyle factors.

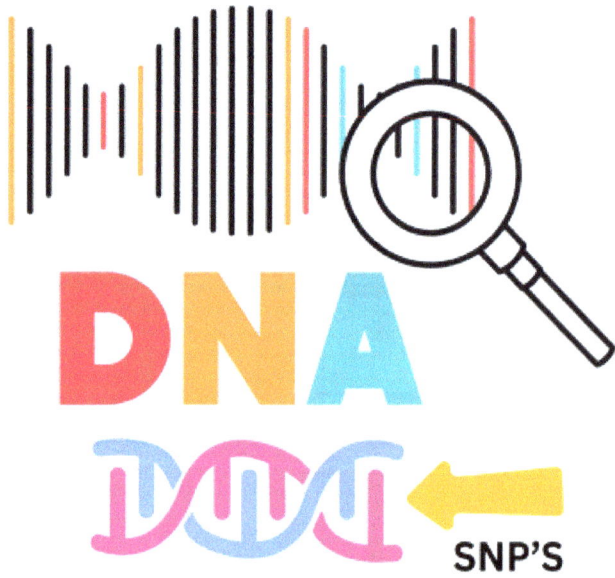

DNA

SNP'S

CHAPTER 8

UNDERSTANDING SNP'S

Understanding single nucleotide polymorphism (SNP) involves grasping the concept of genetic variation at the molecular level. A single nucleotide polymorphism refers to a variation in a DNA sequence where a single nucleotide (A, T, C, or G) is different among individuals within a population.

When a single one of the nucleotides in a gene is other than the normal "letter", it's a variant from the norm called a "Single Nucleotide Polymorphism" or "SNP" (pronounced "snip") for short. Knowing your SNPs can help you determine if a nutrient or food is right for you, as it may have different effects depending on the variant in the gene. Some individuals may be able to tolerate certain foods that cause an adverse reaction in others due to genetic differences.

A SNP can change the function of a gene, and this can have a huge effect on how your body responds to nutrients and other lifestyle factors. This means that each person has their own unique genetic makeup which should be taken into account when creating an individualized nutrition plan. By understanding the implications of your genetic make-up, you can take action to ensure that your diet is tailored to meet your specific needs.

Here are some key points to comprehend about SNPs:

- **BASIC UNIT OF GENETIC VARIATION:** SNPs are the most common type of genetic variation in the human genome. They represent differences in a single DNA building block, or nucleotide, at a specific position in the genome.

- **COMMON OCCURRENCE:** SNPs are widespread throughout the human genome, occurring roughly once in every 300 nucleotides on average. This high frequency makes them valuable markers for studying genetic diversity and population genetics.

- **INFLUENCE ON TRAITS AND DISEASES:** While many SNPs may not have any discernible effect on an individual's traits or health, some can be associated with specific characteristics or susceptibility to certain diseases. These variations can be used in genetic studies to understand the genetic basis of complex traits or diseases.

- **INHERITANCE PATTERNS:** SNPs are inherited from one generation to the next. They can be used in genetic studies to trace familial relationships and ancestry.

- **GENOTYPING TECHNIQUES:** Identifying and analyzing SNPs involve various genotyping techniques, such as DNA sequencing or specialized SNP genotyping assays. These techniques allow researchers to detect and characterize the specific nucleotide variations present in individuals.

- **ROLE IN PERSONALIZED MEDICINE:** Understanding an individual's SNP profile can have implications for personalized medicine. Certain drugs or treatments may be more effective or have different side effects based on an individual's SNP profile.

Understanding these epigenetic processes is critical for studying diseases that involve changes in gene expression, such as cancer and developmental disorders. By comprehending how DNA methylation, histone modification, and noncoding RNA activity influence gene expression, we can develop targeted therapies to treat these conditions effectively.

Moreover, these epigenetic mechanisms have implications for evolution as well. Variations in DNA methylation, histone modification, and noncoding RNA activity contribute to the diversity of life on Earth by causing variations in gene expression between species.

To summarize, DNA methylation, histone modification, and noncoding RNAs play vital roles in regulating gene expression and maintaining proper cellular function. By further exploring these processes, we can expand our understanding of human biology and potentially discover new treatments for a wide array of diseases.

By identifying SNPs associated with certain illnesses or health conditions, you can also be more aware of any potential risks and vulnerabilities. Knowing this information ahead of time can help you take preventive measures to avoid these health issues before they arise. It is also important to note that genetic testing services are not a substitute for professional medical advice, but rather an additional tool for understanding how your body works.

One of the most compelling reasons to consider DNA testing is for personalized healthcare. Your genes hold important information about how your body responds to different treatments and medications. By identifying any genetic variations that may increase your risk for certain conditions or impact your body's ability to process medications, you and your healthcare team can create a customized plan that takes into account your unique genetic makeup. This can lead to more effective treatments and improved health outcomes.

By making small changes in your lifestyle and focusing on taking care of yourself, you can make a big impact on your physical and mental wellbeing. Ultimately, genetic testing can help you live a longer and healthier life.

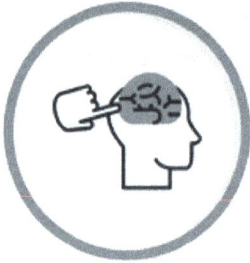
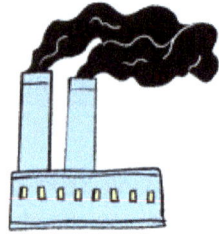
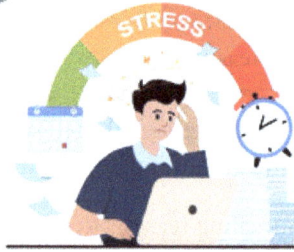
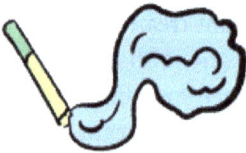
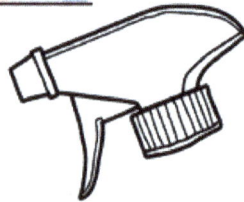

CHAPTER 9

WHAT TRIGGERING EVENTS AFFECT YOUR DNA?

Vaccines have been a topic of controversy for many years, with some people questioning their safety and potential side effects. One common concern is the effect vaccines may have on our DNA.

Because vaccines introduce small amounts of foreign material and or heavy metals into our bodies, some people worry that they could potentially cause harm to our DNA.

I will tell you, DNA is located in the nucleus of our cells, while vaccines generally work outside of the nucleus. However, there is a possibility that some vaccines may cause changes in our DNA. Because this is such a controversial subject I will not expand on this subject. But read my personal story below.

WHAT ARE SOME OTHER TRIGGERS?

"Iatrogenic" refers to conditions or injuries that are unintentionally caused by medical treatment or intervention. The term comes from the Greek words "iatros," meaning "physician," and "genesis," meaning "origin" or "production." Therefore, iatrogenic conditions are essentially those that arise as a result of medical care or procedures.

Medical treatments and interventions are designed to help patients, but sometimes they can lead to unintended side effects or complications. Iatrogenic injuries can occur due to various reasons, including mistakes in medical procedures, adverse reactions to medications, infections acquired in healthcare settings, or other complications arising from medical interventions.

Examples of iatrogenic injuries may include:

- **SURGICAL COMPLICATIONS:** Injuries or complications that occur as a result of surgical procedures. (Dental, anesthesia, pharmaceutical, biologics)

- **MEDICATION SIDE EFFECTS:** Adverse reactions or harm caused by prescribed medications. *Please read your FAQ sheets with every prescription. This is necessary information.

- **INFECTIONS:** Infections acquired during hospital stays or medical treatments. (Bacteria, fungus, viral, mold, yeast, parasites, to mention a few)

- **MISDIAGNOSIS OR MEDICAL ERRORS:** Incorrect diagnoses or mistakes made in medical care that lead to harm.

- **COMPLICATIONS FROM MEDICAL DEVICES:** Problems arising from the use of medical devices or implants.

It's important to note that the vast majority of medical interventions are conducted with the utmost care and expertise, and the benefits typically outweigh the risks. However, the term "iatrogenic" is used to acknowledge and address instances where unintended harm occurs as a result of medical care. Medical professionals and healthcare systems continually strive to minimize iatrogenic risks through improved practices, quality assurance measures, and ongoing education.

There is always a flip side!

If you are not aware of the Vaccine Adverse Event Reporting System, it may be one you want to familiarize yourself with. This system tracks and reports any adverse reactions or side effects from vaccines. While it is important to acknowledge that there can be rare cases of adverse reactions, the benefits of vaccines far outweigh the risks.

I mention this because I ended up with a medical injury six months after a Tdap. I learned I could take the Lot Number of any vaccine and upload it into the www.cdc.gov website to see if the lot was in the "not good" list. It lists all the ingredients and known side effects of each vaccine. My particular Lot Number showed a side effect of "Latent Onset of Type 1 Diabetes in Adults."

This information is not meant to scare or discourage anyone from getting vaccinated, but rather to encourage informed decision-making when it comes to our health. It's always important to do your own research and consult with knowledgeable healthcare professionals before making any decisions.

It is important to know your DNA BLUEPRINT before getting vaccinated, as certain genetic factors and other underlying conditions can affect how your body responds. It is always recommended to consult with a competent healthcare provider before getting vaccinated, especially if you have a compromised immune system or known allergies.

There are five different types of preclinical toxicology study in the evaluation of vaccine safety: single and/or repeat dose, reproductive and developmental, mutagenicity, carcinogenicity, and safety pharmacology. Please do your research for safety concerns and show your doctor your reports.

It's understandable that with so much information out there, it can be overwhelming and confusing to make decisions about conditions put before you. Ultimately, it's important to prioritize our health and make informed choices based on reliable sources of information. While everyone has the right to make their own decisions regarding medical care and toxicology, it is important to approach these topics with an open mind and seek out accurate information.

If you feel you have had an adverse reaction to a vaccine, check the CDC website for the data you're looking for. You will need the LOT NUMBER of the vaccine in question. With this you will gain access to the ingredients and known side effects. https://www.cdc.gov/index.htm

Reporting vaccine-related adverse events to the Vaccine Adverse Event Reporting System https://vaers.hhs.gov/

(VAERS) IS IMPORTANT FOR SEVERAL REASONS:

Early Detection of Safety Concerns: VAERS serves as an early warning system for potential safety concerns related to vaccines. By collecting and analyzing reports of adverse events, public health officials can quickly identify any unusual patterns or trends that may indicate a safety issue.

- **CONTINUOUS MONITORING OF VACCINE SAFETY**: Vaccines go through rigorous testing during development and clinical trials. However, some rare side effects may not be apparent until a vaccine is administered to a larger population. VAERS allows for continuous monitoring of vaccine safety in real-world conditions, helping to ensure ongoing safety and effectiveness.

- **IMPROVING VACCINE SAFETY**: Reporting adverse events to VAERS contributes to the overall understanding of vaccine safety. The information collected helps researchers and public health officials identify areas where improvements can be made in vaccine development and administration. This continuous feedback loop is crucial for refining and enhancing vaccine safety protocols.

- **PUBLIC CONFIDENCE:** Transparency in reporting and addressing vaccine-related adverse events enhances public confidence in vaccination programs. When individuals see that their concerns are taken seriously and that there is a system in place to monitor and investigate adverse events, it can build trust in the vaccination process.

- **EDUCATIONAL PURPOSES:** VAERS data is used for educational purposes to inform healthcare providers, researchers, and the public about the safety profile of vaccines. This information helps healthcare professionals make informed decisions and provide accurate information to their patients.

It's important to note that while VAERS is a valuable tool for monitoring vaccine safety, the reported events are not always confirmed to be directly caused by vaccines. VAERS collects data on any adverse events that occur after vaccination, whether or not they are related to the vaccine. This inclusive reporting approach ensures that all potential concerns are investigated thoroughly.

If someone experiences an adverse event after vaccination, healthcare professionals and individuals are encouraged to report it to VAERS. Reporting can be done online, and the information provided contributes to the ongoing efforts to maintain the safety of vaccines.

*Talk to your healthcare provider about any concerns or questions you may have.

*Stay informed about current outbreaks and recommended vaccinations from reliable sources such as the CDC. **DO YOUR RESEARCH!**

Let's work together to promote and prioritize public health.

In terms of potential reactions to medications or vaccines, epigenetic testing can be beneficial. Some individuals may have genetic variations that impact how their bodies metabolize certain drugs, leading to adverse reactions or side effects. By identifying these variations beforehand, healthcare professionals can adjust doses or choose alternative treatments to avoid potential negative effects. This can also help prevent unnecessary trial and error with different medications, saving time and money for both the patient and their healthcare provider.

There are plenty of articles available for you to research. There were a few that were of particular concern to me after twenty years of active duty time in the U.S. Air Force. After the medical injury in 2019, I have always wondered if it was the ingredients that was the straw that broke the camel's back? Or is that what put my body in an over-immunological response to where it attacked my pancreas? The answers may never be fully clear, but with DNA testing, you can get a better understanding of your genetic predispositions and potential reactions to certain medications or vaccines.

Military vaccinations: https://www.ncbi.nlm.nih.gov/books/NBK222854/

What Triggering Events Affect Your DNA?

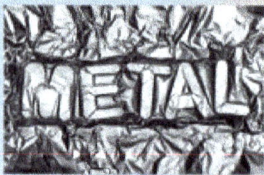

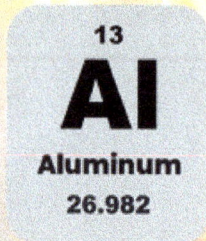

13
Al
Aluminum
26.982

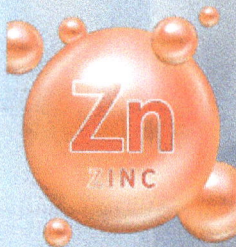

Zn
ZINC

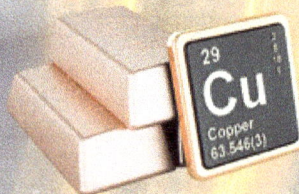

29
Cu
Copper
63.546(3)

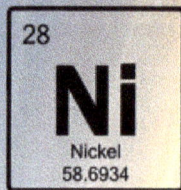

28
Ni
Nickel
58.6934

CHAPTER 10

UNVEILING THE DANGERS OF HEAVY METAL POISONING

I n the intricate tapestry of health, heavy metal poisoning emerges as a formidable adversary, its insidious presence concealed within microscopic molecules that silently infiltrate the human body following exposure. These minuscule agents, composed of various metals, forge a perilous connection with our cells, obstructing their vital functions and unleashing a cascade of symptoms that, if left untreated, could pose life-threatening consequences.

The roster of metals capable of inducing heavy metal poisoning reads like a chilling inventory of toxic intruders. Among them, some of the most notorious culprits include:

- **LEAD:** Stealthily infiltrating through avenues such as contaminated water flowing through lead pipes, as well as lurking in batteries, paint, gasoline, and construction materials.

- **MERCURY:** A lurking threat found in liquid form within thermometers, lightbulbs, dental amalgam ("silver") fillings, batteries, seafood, and even topical antiseptics.

- **ARSENIC:** Posing a danger through various channels like topical creams, herbicides, insecticides, pesticides, fungicides, paints, enamels, glass, contaminated water, seafood, and algae.

- **CADMIUM:** Stealthily making its way into the body through cigarette smoke, metal plating, and batteries.

- **THALLIUM:** An elusive menace present in rodenticides, pesticides, and even fireworks.

This chapter unravels the intricate web of heavy metal toxicity, shedding light on the sources and consequences of exposure to these malevolent substances. As we delve into the realm of heavy metal poisoning, it becomes evident that awareness and understanding are crucial shields against its potentially dire effects on human health.

Heavy metal toxicity refers to the accumulation of excessive amounts of certain metals in the body, which can lead to adverse health effects. Different heavy metals can have varying toxicities, and the specific symptoms and impacts depend on the type of metal, the level of exposure, and individual factors. Some common heavy metals associated with toxicity include lead, mercury, arsenic, cadmium, and chromium.

HERE ARE GENERAL EFFECTS OF HEAVY METAL TOXICITY ON THE BODY:

- **NEUROLOGICAL EFFECTS:** Many heavy metals have neurotoxic effects, particularly lead and mercury. Exposure to these metals can lead to cognitive impairments, memory loss, mood changes, and difficulty concentrating. In children, lead exposure is particularly concerning as it can impact cognitive development.

- **CARDIOVASCULAR EFFECTS:** Some heavy metals, such as lead and cadmium, have been associated with cardiovascular problems. They can contribute to high blood pressure, atherosclerosis, and an increased risk of heart disease.

- **RENAL (KIDNEY) EFFECTS:** Heavy metals like cadmium and lead can accumulate in the kidneys, leading to kidney damage and dysfunction over time. Chronic exposure may result in kidney disease.

- **RESPIRATORY ISSUES:** Inhalation of certain heavy metals, such as cadmium and lead, can cause respiratory problems. Exposure to these metals in occupational settings or through environmental pollution can lead to lung damage and respiratory disorders.

- **GASTROINTESTINAL EFFECTS:** Ingesting heavy metals, either through contaminated food or water, can lead to gastrointestinal issues. Symptoms may include nausea, vomiting, abdominal pain, and diarrhea.

- **HEPATIC (LIVER) EFFECTS:** Some heavy metals, like cadmium, can accumulate in the liver and contribute to liver damage. Chronic exposure may lead to liver disease.

- **REPRODUCTIVE AND DEVELOPMENTAL EFFECTS:** Certain heavy metals, including lead and mercury, can have adverse effects on reproductive health and fetal development. Pregnant women exposed to high levels of these metals may face an increased risk of developmental issues in their children.

- **SKIN ISSUES:** Contact with certain heavy metals can cause skin irritation and dermatitis. For example, exposure to nickel or chromium compounds can lead to skin allergies.

It's important to note that the severity of the effects depends on factors such as the duration and intensity of exposure, individual susceptibility, and the type of heavy metal involved. Chronic exposure to low levels of heavy metals over an extended period is a common concern, and preventive measures, such as reducing environmental exposure and occupational safety measures, are essential to minimize the risk of toxicity. If someone suspects heavy metal exposure or toxicity, they should seek medical attention for evaluation and appropriate management.

A heavy metal detoxification will help to eliminate the excess heavy metals from the body and reduce their potential harmful effects. This process involves removing heavy metals from tissues, organs, and cells through various methods such as chelation therapy, sauna therapy, and dietary changes. Chelation therapy is a medical procedure that involves administering chelating agents (substances that bind to heavy metals) either orally or intravenously to assist in the elimination of toxic metals from the body.

Additionally, some foods and supplements can help support the detoxification process, including foods rich in antioxidants like fruits and vegetables, as well as mineral-rich foods such as leafy greens and seaweed. It's essential to consult with a healthcare professional before starting any detoxification program, especially if there are underlying health conditions or allergies.

Sauna therapy is another method commonly used for detoxification. Sweating helps to eliminate toxins from the body, and saunas can provide a more intense sweat than exercise alone. They also offer other benefits such as relaxation and improved circulation.

Along with these methods, making dietary changes can also aid in the detoxification process. This includes reducing intake of processed foods, refined sugars, and alcohol while increasing consumption of whole foods like lean proteins, healthy fats, and complex carbohydrates.

It's crucial to note that the body has its own natural detoxification processes through organs such as the liver, kidneys, and skin. These organs work together to filter out toxins from the body constantly. However, due to environmental factors and our modern diets high in chemicals and additives, our bodies may need a little extra help in detoxifying. Especially if you have an active gene that does not allow your body to detox properly. For instance, reduced NRF2 expression might hinder the body's ability to detoxify substances leading to oxidative stress.

One popular method is through the use of detox diets or cleanses. These programs involve eliminating certain food groups and consuming specific foods or drinks for a set period. Some proponents claim that these diets can help remove toxins from the body, improve digestion, and boost energy levels.

However, it's important to approach these diets with caution as they often lack scientific evidence to support their claims. Plus, restricting certain food groups can lead to nutrient deficiencies and potential negative side effects. It's always best to consult with a healthcare professional before starting any type of detox program.

Another natural way to support the body's detoxification process is by staying hydrated. Drinking plenty of water helps flush out toxins. Hydrogenated water and herbal teas are also beneficial in aiding the body's natural detoxification process.

In addition, incorporating more whole foods into your diet, such as fruits and vegetables, can provide essential vitamins and minerals to support overall health. Choosing organic options when possible can also help reduce exposure to toxins found in pesticides and other chemicals commonly used in conventional farming.

Exercise is another key component in supporting the body's detoxification process. Sweating helps release toxins through the skin, while physical activity stimulates circulation and improves lymphatic function. Yoga, in particular, is known for its detoxifying benefits due to its focus on deep breathing exercises and twisting poses that help stimulate digestion and improve blood flow.

Lastly, managing stress levels is crucial for a healthy body and mind. Chronic stress can lead to inflammation and weakening of the immune system, making it more difficult for the body to detox-ify properly. Incorporating stress-reducing activities such as medi-tation, mindfulness practices, or regular relaxation techniques can greatly support the body's natural detoxification process.

Overall, adopting healthy lifestyle habits such as eating a nutri-ent-rich diet, staying physically active, and managing stress is key in supporting our body's detoxification process. By consistently fueling our bodies with nourishing foods and engaging in regular self-care practices, we can help optimize our natural detoxification pathways and promote overall well-being. Remember to always listen to your body's needs and make adjustments accordingly. With these simple steps, you can help support your body's natural ability to detoxify and thrive.

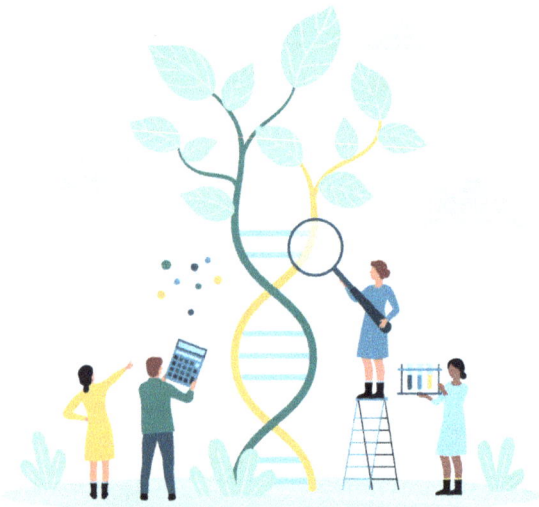

Defining The Genes

CHAPTER 11

DEFINING THE GENES

Before I break down the specific genes which are in the nutrigenomic testing, I want to discuss Autophagy, a lysosome-dependent degradation pathway.

Autophagy is a cellular process that involves the degradation and recycling of damaged or unnecessary cellular components, such as organelles and proteins. It is a vital mechanism for maintaining cellular homeostasis and responding to various stressors, including starvation, oxidative stress, and DNA damage. The term "autophagy" is derived from the Greek words "auto" (self) and "phagy" (eating), reflecting the process by which cells consume their own components.

Autophagy is like a cellular cleanup crew that helps keep our cells healthy. When our cells face stress, like from starvation or damage to their DNA (the genetic material), autophagy kicks in.

Imagine autophagy as a janitorial service in our cells. When there's a mess, like damaged organelles or proteins, autophagy comes in to clean up. It puts the damaged stuff in a kind of cellular trash bag called an autophagosome, which then gets sent to the cell's trash disposal unit, the lysosome. There, everything gets broken down into reusable parts.

Autophagy is especially important when it comes to DNA damage. If there's a problem with the genetic instructions inside the cell, autophagy helps by getting rid of the damaged parts. It's like a repair and recycling system for the cell's genetic material.

Also, autophagy is good at keeping the powerhouses of the cell, called mitochondria, in good shape. Mitochondria have their own DNA, and if they get damaged, it can be bad for the cell. Autophagy steps in to remove and recycle these damaged mitochondria, ensuring the cell stays healthy. It is a cellular process that helps regulate cell fate after DNA damage and is essential for maintaining genomic integrity,

Time to define the actionable SNP's.

APOB_RS693* (APOLIPOPROTEIN B) - HEALTHY LIPID SUPPORT

The ApoB_rs693 Gene regulates the main protein component of LDL - supporting healthy cholesterol.

Are you aware of the ApoB gene and its role in maintaining a healthy heart? This gene plays a vital role in supporting cardiovascular health by ensuring that cholesterol levels remain within the normal range.

Understanding the Significance of the ApoB Gene:

Cholesterol is transported in the bloodstream via lipoproteins, namely low-density lipoprotein (LDL) and high-density lipoprotein (HDL). The ApoB gene regulates the production of apolipoprotein B (ApoB), the main protein component of LDL. In fact, LDL formation is impossible without ApoB. Maintaining healthy LDL levels has been associated with better cardiovascular health, as indicated by research illustrating an inverse connection between ApoB levels and heart health.

Supporting Individuals with the ApoB Gene SNP:

Individuals with a single nucleotide polymorphism (SNP) in the ApoB gene can benefit from supplementation with ingredients that help maintain ApoB production, retain healthy cholesterol levels, and support cardiovascular health.

The Relationship Between ApoB_rs693 Gene and Coronary Artery Disease (CAD):

For those with cholesterol issues, it is essential to understand the impact of the ApoB_rs693 gene on the risk of CAD. This gene encodes apolipoprotein B-100, a major lipoprotein involved in delivering cholesterol to tissues. Carrying the ApoB_rs693 SNP has been linked to increased levels of total cholesterol, LDL cholesterol, and a higher risk of developing CAD.

Managing Cholesterol Levels:

Reducing cholesterol and LDL-C levels is crucial for ApoB_rs693 carriers. Adopting a balanced diet, engaging in regular physical activity, and maintaining a healthy weight can help achieve this. Specific dietary recommendations include limiting saturated fats, trans fats, and cholesterol as well as increasing fiber intake. Intermittent fasting and following a Mediterranean diet have been found to be beneficial.

Take Control of Your Heart Health:

APoB_rs693 carriers should focus on reducing cholesterol and LDL-C levels. A person with this gene cannot burn bad fats unless they take in good fats. This person may have fat in the hips, thighs, and leg area.

*A white paper in April 2022 stated statin drugs really didn't help cholesterol. Less than 8-10% of cholesterol comes from diet.

Dietary Recommendations to Support the ApoB Gene:

1. **GREEN TEA EXTRACT:** Clinical trials have shown that supplementing with green tea catechins can help maintain healthy LDL levels in adults. Additionally, green tea catechins have been found to reduce ApoB activity.

2. **GRAPE SKIN EXTRACT:** In vitro studies have demonstrated that the polyphenols in red wine can help decrease ApoB levels.

3. **POMEGRANATE EXTRACT:** Research indicates that consuming pomegranate juice promotes cardiovascular health and increases the activity of serum paraoxonase, which protects against lipid peroxidation.

4. **ARTICHOKE EXTRACT:** Well-documented for its ability to support cholesterol levels and positively modulate endothelial function, artichoke extract contributes to a healthy heart and vascular system.

Ideally, a person should focus on eating whole grains, fruits, vegetables, nuts, beans and legumes. These foods are packed with dietary fiber, antioxidants, vitamins and minerals that can help keep cholesterol levels in check. Eating fish twice a week is also beneficial as it contains omega-3 fatty acids which have been shown to reduce the risk of heart disease.

Limit the following:

- Red meat and processed meats like sausages, bacon, etc.,
- Dairy products such as cream and cheese that are high in saturated fat,
- Fried foods
- Sugary drinks and snacks like soda, candy and cakes

ATP5C1_RS1244414* MITOCHONDRIAL ATP SYNTHASE - MITOCHONDRIAL FUNCTION

Important for energy production in the cell. Think of it as batteries. Cell regeneration and energy necessary to fuel our cellular daily functions.

Discover the Importance and Impact of the ATP5C1 Gene on Your Energy Levels

The ATP5C1 gene plays a crucial role in energy production within your cells. It encodes the gamma subunit of the mitochondrial ATP synthase enzyme, which is responsible for producing ATP. This gene is part of complex V in the mitochondrial respiratory chain.

If you have a variant of the ATP5C1 gene, your mitochondria may not be functioning properly. This can lead to fatigue, low energy, difficulty concentrating, and memory problems. In severe cases, it can even result in muscle pain, vision and hearing problems, heart issues, and other serious ailments.

But don't worry, there are ways to support and improve your mitochondrial function. One effective method is through dietary recommendations. Incorporating certain ingredients into your diet can support your mitochondria and enhance cellular energy.

Consider adding PQQ (Pyrroloquinoline Quinone) to your routine. Known for increasing the number and efficiency of mitochondria, PQQ can be a valuable addition to your supplement plan.

Ubiquinone and ubiquinol, also known as CoQ10, are major antioxidants that not only support cardiovascular health but also contribute to cellular energy. As we age, the production of CoQ10 decreases, making supplementation even more important. Different dosages of ubiquinone and ubiquinol are available, so choose the one that fits your needs.

CoQ10 is a major antioxidant that supports cardiovascular health and is important for cellular energy. As we age, production of CoQ10 levels decreases. Depending on the number of gene variants your DNA has the follow may be needed: Green (0 copies) 50 mg ubiquinone • Yellow (single copy): 25 mg ubiquinone and 25 mg ubiquinol • Red (Double copy): 50 mg ubiquinol

Alpha Lipoic Acid is another antioxidant that aids in the restoration of certain vitamin levels and helps break down carbohydrates. It can also be beneficial for stabilizing blood sugar levels. Remember, individuals with a genetic variant in the ATP5C1 gene can benefit from supplementation with ingredients that support mitochondrial function and cellular energy.

In addition to dietary recommendations, lifestyle changes can also have a positive impact on your mitochondrial health. Incorporating intermittent fasting, 8-12 hours, and low-carbohydrate diets has been found to be beneficial for individuals with mitochondrial diseases. These approaches optimize the body's energy usage and reduce inflammation, ultimately improving symptoms. Exercise and adequate rest are essential for managing mitochondrial disease. Physical activity can improve mobility, energy efficiency, and reduce fatigue associated with mitochondrial diseases. Getting enough sleep is vital for restorative processes in the body and can contribute to better overall health. It will help to remove cellular waste.

To further support your mitochondrial health, aim for a pH range of 7-7.2, which is slightly alkaline. Avoiding fried and processed foods and consuming more anti-inflammatory fruits and vegetables, especially those that are green, purple, and blue, can also make a difference.

By taking appropriate care and making the right choices, you can live a full and productive life, even with mitochondrial disease.

CRP_RS1205* (C-REACTIVE PROTEIN) - HEALTHY INFLAMMATORY RESPONSE

The CRP_rs1205 gene variant has been linked to the body's production of C-reactive protein (CRP), which is a marker for inflammation in the body. However, this does not necessarily mean that individuals with this gene variant will develop health conditions related to inflammation.

It balances out too little or too much inflammation. CRP increases during an acute inflammatory response. Inflammation can be caused by various factors such as an unhealthy diet, smoking, lack of exercise, and stress. By making small changes in our lifestyle, we can reduce the level of inflammation in our bodies and improve overall health.

There are many lifestyle changes that can help decrease chronic inflammation in the body. Incorporating regular exercise, stress management techniques, and quitting smoking and limiting alcohol consumption can all contribute to reducing inflammation and improving overall health. Smoking has been linked to increased inflammation and can also hinder the body's ability to heal itself. Alcohol, on the other hand, can cause gut dysbiosis and leaky gut, which can increase inflammation.

In addition to exercise, maintaining a healthy diet is crucial in reducing inflammation. Foods rich in antioxidants, omega-3 fatty acids, and polyphenols have been shown to have anti-inflammatory properties. These include fruits and vegetables, whole grains, nuts and seeds, fatty fish like salmon and tuna, and green tea. So don't wait any longer. Start making small changes today for big benefits tomorrow!

We are not done yet!

A person with the CRP_rs1205 gene variant would have swollen inflammation in all joints, and may need medication to balance out their inflammatory response.

The human body needs certain nutrients for health. Eating a balanced and varied diet full of whole foods and limiting or avoiding processed foods is important for optimal health.

They may also experience chronic fatigue, abdominal pain, and headaches. Other symptoms of this gene variant include depression, anxiety, insomnia, memory problems, dizziness, skin rashes, and numbness in the hands and feet. In extreme cases, this gene variant can cause an increased risk for autoimmune diseases such as Lupus and Rheumatoid Arthritis. Long-term treatment for this gene mutation usually involves lifestyle changes, such as regular exercise and relaxation techniques, as well as medications to reduce inflammation and improve sleep quality. In some cases, physical therapy may be recommended to help with symptoms. A person with the CRP_rs1205 gene variant should monitor their diet and supplement intake to ensure that their body is getting all the required nutrients.

It is important to note that while the CRP_rs1205 gene variant has been linked to certain health conditions, it is not a guarantee of any illness. There are numerous other factors, such as lifestyle and family history, that contribute to an individual's overall health. It is best to do 20-30 minutes of walking at least 2-3 times per week. Have C-reactive protein blood checks as the inflammation weakens the immune system. Have your doctor test you 2x a year.

Try a Mediterranean diet with good healthy fats is key. Eat more anti-inflammatory food like olive oil, green leafy vegetables.

CYP11B2_RS1799998* (HEALTHY BLOOD PRESSURE)

Responsible for maintaining blood pressure in normal ranges, essential for a healthy heart. It also supports healthy adrenals.

Unlock the Secrets to Maintaining Healthy Blood Pressure

Are you struggling to keep your blood pressure in check? Look no further! The CYP11B2 gene is here to help. This incredible gene plays a vital role in maintaining blood pressure within the normal range, ensuring a healthy heart.

Why is the CYP11B2 Gene Important?

Maintaining a healthy heart starts with controlling your blood pressure. The CYP11B2 gene produces an enzyme called aldosterone synthase, which is crucial for the proper balance of salt and fluid in your body. By supporting healthy blood pressure levels, this gene contributes to overall cardiovascular health.

Dietary Recommendations for Maximizing the Potential of the CYP11B2 Gene

Want to enhance the benefits of the CYP11B2 gene? Try these powerful ingredients that have been scientifically proven to maintain blood pressure levels within the normal range and support cardiovascular health:

- **HAWTHORN BERRY EXTRACT:** Strengthen your heart function and reinforce healthy blood pressure and cholesterol levels with this natural cardiotonic.

- **MAGNESIUM AND POTASSIUM:** These essential minerals are known to support healthy blood pressure levels.

- **VITAMIN C AND GARLIC POWDER:** These ingredients help maintain blood pressure within the normal range and support overall cardiovascular health.

Take Control of Your Health

If you have the CYP11B2_rs1799998 variant, don't worry! With a few simple lifestyle changes, you can effectively manage your blood pressure and overall health. Here are some tips to get you started:

- **STAY ACTIVE:** Regular exercise, such as walking or yoga, can help keep your blood pressure in check.

- **EAT RIGHT:** A healthy diet rich in fruits and vegetables can help balance hormones and support your cardiovascular health.

- **REDUCE STRESS:** Practice stress-relieving activities like meditation, deep breathing exercises, or prayer.

- **HYDRATE, HYDRATE, HYDRATE:** Drinking plenty of water is essential for regulating hormones and flushing out toxins.

- **SLEEP WELL:** Good sleep is crucial for overall health, so aim for at least 7-8 hours of quality sleep each night.

Stay Informed, Stay Healthy.

Break Free from the Grip of Unhealthy Blood Pressure

Kick caffeine to the curb, steer clear of high-sodium processed foods, and limit alcohol intake. With these simple tips, you can take control of your health and break free from the limitations of unhealthy blood pressure.

Take control of your blood pressure and overall well-being with these essential tips. Maintain a healthy lifestyle through regular exercise, a nutritious diet, and stress reduction techniques. Stay vigilant by monitoring your blood pressure and documenting any changes. Collaborate with your healthcare provider to find the best treatment plan for your unique needs. Don't forget to discuss any other health conditions that might be impacted by this variant. Stay informed about the latest research to make informed health-care decisions.

Sleep well to safeguard your health. Inadequate sleep has been linked to increased medical risks. Manage stress effectively with activities like yoga, Tai Chi, walking, meditation, deep breathing exercises, or prayer. Enhance hormone balance and support over-all health with a diet rich in fruits and vegetables. And don't forget to stay hydrated! Water is crucial for regulating hormones, reducing fatigue, and flushing out toxins.

Regular medical checkups are essential to monitor hormone levels and adjust medications or treatments as needed. Seek support from a mental health professional if you're feeling overwhelmed or experiencing anxiety related to the variant. They can help you navigate the challenges and provide valuable assistance.

Effort is required to manage the CYP11B1 variant. Avoid caffeine, as it dehydrates the body and increases blood pressure. Watch out for potential symptoms such as leg swelling, impaired night vision while driving, digestive issues, fatigue, adrenal fatigue, kidney stress, ringing in the ears, and low magnesium levels. Limit your intake of table salt, processed foods high in sodium, and alcohol. Take charge of your health and live your best life.

Knowledge is power when it comes to managing the CYP11B2 variant. Keep up to date with the latest research, consult with your healthcare provider regularly, and consider seeking the support of a mental health professional if needed. By taking these proactive steps, you can thrive with the CYP11B2_rs1799998 variant and live a healthy, fulfilled life.

MTHFR_RS1801133* (METHYLENE TETRAHYDROFOLATE REDUCTASE) - HOMOCYSTEINE FOLATE (VARIANT C677T)

Responsible for folic acid to folate conversion.

In the intricate landscape of our genetic code, the MTHFR_rs1801133* gene takes center stage as a master conductor. At its core, this gene plays a pivotal role in the conversion of folic acid, the synthetic form of folate, into its natural and bioactive counterpart—folate. This conversion is akin to the ignition of fuel, a crucial step that propels energy into the cells. Folate, a B-vitamin, emerges as a fundamental component for numerous biological processes within our body.

Fueling Cellular Energy:

Picture folate as the gasoline that powers the engine of cellular energy. Through its enzymatic prowess, it ensures a seamless transformation, allowing folate to serve as a potent source of energy for our cells. This process isn't just a biochemical nuance; it is the very essence of vitality at the cellular level.

The impact of this gene extends far beyond a singular reaction. This gene serves as the gateway to a vast network of approximately 250 biochemical reactions in the body. From DNA synthesis and repair to neurotransmitter production, It exerts its influence, shaping the very foundation of our health and well-being.

But what happens when this gene is not functioning optimally? When MTHFR_rs1801133* is mutated, our body's ability to utilize folate is impaired. This can lead to a deficiency in cellular energy production and an array of health issues.

Potential Effects of MTHFR_rs1801133* Mutations:

1. **REDUCED FOLATE LEVELS:** Without proper MTHFR_rs1801133* function, folate cannot be converted into its active form, 5-MTHF. This leads to reduced levels of 5-MTHF in the body, which is essential for DNA synthesis and repair. Low levels of 5-MTHF have been linked to birth defects, cardiovascular diseases, and neurological disorders.

2. **INCREASED RISK OF MENTAL HEALTH ISSUES:** Studies have shown that individuals with this mutation are more likely to develop mental health disorders such as depression, anxiety, and bipolar disorder. This is because 5-MTHF plays a crucial role in the production of neurotransmitters like serotonin and dopamine, which regulate our mood and emotions.

3. **IMPAIRED DETOXIFICATION:** The MTHFR_rs1801133* gene also helps in the detoxification process by converting homocysteine to methionine. A mutation in this gene can lead to elevated levels of homocysteine, which has been linked to an

increased risk of cardiovascular diseases, Alzheimer's disease, and dementia.

4. **COMPLICATIONS DURING PREGNANCY:** Pregnant women with MTHFR_rs1801133* mutations are at a higher risk of developing complications such as preeclampsia, recurrent miscarriages, and neural tube defects in their babies. This is because the gene plays an essential role in the development of the baby's brain and spinal cord.

5. **IMPACT ON FOLATE METABOLISM:** Folate is an essential vitamin that our bodies need for DNA synthesis and repair, red blood cell production, and healthy fetal development. MTHFR_rs1801133* mutations can lead to impaired folate metabolism, which can cause deficiencies in this vital nutrient.

6. **DIETARY CHANGES CAN HELP:** While we cannot change our gene mutation, we can make dietary changes to support healthy folate metabolism and minimize the risks associated with MTHFR_rs1801133* mutations. This includes increasing our intake of folate-rich foods such as leafy green vegetables, legumes, citrus fruits, and fortified grains. It is also recommended to take a prenatal vitamin with folic acid to ensure adequate levels of this crucial nutrient.

7. **CONSULTATION WITH A HEALTHCARE PROVIDER:** If you are pregnant or planning to become pregnant and have the MTHFR_rs1801133* mutation, it is essential to consult with your healthcare provider. They can provide personalized guidance on managing your condition and reducing potential risks for both you and your baby.

8. **IMPORTANCE OF PRENATAL TESTING:** Prenatal testing for genetic mutations, including MTHFR_rs1801133*, can help identify any potential risks for pregnancy complications. This can include screening for neural tube defects and other birth

defects associated with low folate levels. It is important to discuss these options with your healthcare provider.

9. **SEEKING SUPPORT:** Coping with a genetic mutation during pregnancy can be overwhelming, and seeking support from others who are going through a similar experience can be beneficial. There are online communities and support groups available for individuals with this mutation, providing a space to share experiences, ask questions, and find support.

10. **CONCLUSION:** Being aware of the MTHFR_rs1801133* mutation and its potential effects on pregnancy health is crucial for expecting mothers. By following these recommended steps and working closely with your healthcare provider, you can ensure the best possible outcome for you and your baby. Remember, knowledge is power, and being proactive about your health during pregnancy can make all the difference. Don't hesitate to reach out for support and guidance throughout your journey. We wish you a happy and healthy pregnancy!

Explore the dietary recommendations and lifestyle adjustments that can help you manage your homocysteine levels and support cardiovascular health.

Maximize the Benefits of the MTHFR Gene:

- **DIETARY RECOMMENDATIONS:** Tailor your diet to support your MTHFR gene. Incorporate foods rich in B vitamins, such as beef, poultry, fatty fish, leafy greens, fresh fruits, and eggs. Avoid excess alcohol consumption, limiting intake to 2 drinks per day for men and 1 drink per day for women.

- **VISIT YOUR HEALTHCARE PROVIDER:** Regularly check in with your healthcare provider to monitor your homocysteine, folate, b12, and CBC levels through blood work. Stay proactive in managing your health.

- **SUPPLEMENT SUPPORT:** Consider supplementation with nutrients like trimethylglycine (TMG), choline bitartrate, and reduced folate (5-methyltetrahydrofolic acid) to maintain healthy homocysteine levels and overall cardiovascular health.

Lifestyle Adjustments for Optimal Results:

1. **AVOID SYNTHETIC FOLIC ACID:** Synthetic folic acid can have a detrimental effect on individuals with the MTHFR gene variant. Stay away from breads, grains, and processed foods fortified with synthetic B vitamins. Only opt for methylated B vitamins.

2. **PRIORITIZE SLEEP:** Address any sleep issues by ensuring you get 7-9 hours of quality sleep per day. Sleep is essential for your overall well-being and can help regulate your neurotransmitters.

3. **HYDRATION AND DETOXIFICATION:** Hydrate your body to facilitate the elimination of toxins. Detoxification is crucial for healing. Methylation is a significant concern for folate metabolism. This includes consuming more foods high in folate, such as leafy greens, beans, and fortified grains. It is also recommended to take a prenatal vitamin with folic acid to ensure proper nutrient intake during pregnancy.

4. **IMPORTANCE OF GENETIC TESTING:** If you have a family history of MTHFR_rs1801133* mutations or have experienced complications during previous pregnancies, that can be addressed by consuming a nutrient-rich, whole foods diet. Avoid high-fructose corn syrup, artificial sweeteners, hydrogenated oils, and GMO foods.

Empower yourself with the knowledge of your MTHFR gene and take charge of your health. By making simple dietary and lifestyle adjustments, you can support your body's natural processes and enhance your overall well-being.

With the right lifestyle choices and a little effort, you can maintain healthy gut flora and overall good health!

MTHFR_RS1801131* (METHYLENE TETRAHYDROFOLATE REDUCTASE) - HOMOCYSTEINE FOLATE (VARIANT A1298C)

Navigating the Homocysteine Pathway to Cardiovascular Wellness

Embarking on the journey of understanding our genetic code, the MTHFR gene emerges as a key orchestrator sharing a fundamental role in the genetic regulation of homocysteine, showcasing its significance in maintaining cardiovascular health through the intricate conversion of folic acid.

While MTHFR_rs1801131* and MTHFR_rs1801133* share similarities in their role as key players in homocysteine regulation, they differ in certain genetic aspects. Here are the distinctions between the two:

Genetic Location:

MTHFR_rs1801131* and MTHFR_rs1801133* represent different genetic variants located at distinct positions on the MTHFR gene. Each variant is characterized by a specific alteration in the DNA sequence, influencing the enzyme's structure and function.

Specific Genetic Variants:

These genes carry different specific genetic variants or Single Nucleotide Polymorphisms (SNPs). The variations in the DNA sequence at these specific positions can affect the enzymatic activity of MTHFR, potentially influencing homocysteine metabolism.

Enzyme Activity Impact:

The specific genetic variants may have different effects on the enzyme's activity. Some variants may result in reduced enzyme efficiency, impacting the conversion of folic acid to folate and, consequently, homocysteine regulation.

Population Frequencies:

The prevalence of these genetic variants can vary among populations. Different ethnic groups may exhibit distinct frequencies of variants, contributing to variations in how individuals metabolize folate and manage homocysteine levels.

Clinical Associations:

Research has explored associations between these genetic variants and various health conditions. Studies have investigated potential links between specific MTHFR_rs1801131* or MTHFR_rs1801133* variants and conditions such as cardiovascular diseases, neural tube defects, and other health outcomes. The nature and strength of these associations can differ between the two variants.

Clinical Implications:

The clinical significance of MTHFR_rs1801131* and MTHFR_rs1801133* may vary based on their specific genetic variants. Certain variants may be associated with an increased risk of certain health conditions, while others may not have a significant impact.

While both MTHFR_rs1801131* and MTHFR_rs1801133* contribute to homocysteine regulation, their differences lie in the specific genetic variants they represent, their impact on enzyme activity, population frequencies, associations with health conditions, and clinical implications. Understanding these distinctions is crucial for personalized healthcare and genetic risk assessment.

By following the steps above, you can stay on track with managing your MTHFR mutation and achieving optimal health. Remember to keep an open dialogue with your doctor about any changes in your health or symptoms that could be related to your MTHFR mutation. With the right care, you'll stay healthy and strong. Good luck!

MTRR_RS1801394* (METHIONINE SYNTHASE REDUCTASE) - HOMOCYSTEINE HEALTHY HEART FORMULA

Decoding the MTRR Gene: Guardian of Cardiovascular Health

In the intricate language of DNA, the MTRR gene emerges as a silent hero, wielding the power to safeguard cardiovascular health. Let's unravel the mysteries surrounding this genetic guardian and explore the profound impact it has on our well-being.

Unveiling the Purpose of MTRR

Why is the MTRR gene important? Homocysteine, a metabolite of the amino acid methionine, can be detrimental to cardiovascular health. The MTRR enzyme helps to control homocysteine levels by converting it back into methionine. Research has shown that maintaining healthy homocysteine levels is crucial for preserving cardiovascular health.

Homocysteine, though a natural byproduct of methionine metabolism, demands careful oversight. The MTRR enzyme steps into this role, ensuring that homocysteine levels are kept in check. Research underscores the significance of maintaining a delicate balance, as elevated homocysteine levels can pose risks to cardiovascular well-being.

Nourishing the MTRR Gene: Dietary Recommendations

Understanding the importance of the MTRR gene, especially in the presence of a Single Nucleotide Polymorphism (SNP), prompts strategic dietary interventions. The MTRR SNP finds support in a carefully curated combination of ingredients designed to maintain healthy homocysteine levels and bolster overall cardiovascular health.

Key Dietary Recommendations:

1. **B VITAMINS:**
   Vitamins B2, B6, folate, and B12 join forces to synergistically aid the body in processing homocysteine efficiently.

2. **NIACIN (VITAMIN B3):**
   A stalwart in cardioprotection, Niacin has been trusted for decades for its overall cardiovascular benefits.

3. **TRIMETHYLGLYCINE (TMG OR BETAINE):**
   A key compound supporting the conversion of homocysteine to methionine, enhancing the activity of B Vitamins in the process.

4. **DONG QUAI EXTRACT:**
   Hailing from Chinese herbal traditions, Dong Quai strengthens vital organs, fortifies the liver, and aids in balancing homocysteine levels through improved oxygen utilization and enhanced glutathione enzyme activity.

5. **ZINC:**
   Acting as a cofactor alongside Vitamin B6, Zinc plays a crucial role in the conversion of homocysteine to methionine.

Individuals with an MTRR gene SNP stand to benefit from supplementation with these ingredients, aiming to:

• Manage homocysteine levels effectively.

• Support the conversion of homocysteine to methionine.

• Enhance overall cardiovascular health.

In the intricate tapestry of genes and nutrition, the MTRR gene emerges as a key player, influencing our cardiovascular symphony. As we decode its nuances, we gain insights that empower us to make informed dietary choices, embracing a path of wellness guided by the wisdom embedded in our DNA.

NQ01_RS1800566* (COENZYME Q10 REDUCTASE) - COQ10 ENERGY

Purpose of NQ01

The NQ01 gene plays a pivotal role in dictating whether the body utilizes ubiquinone or ubiquinol, the two forms of CoQ10. This genetic determinant is crucial in the process of eliminating free radicals and facilitating cellular energy production within the body.

The Importance of NQ01

CoQ10 stands out as a potent antioxidant essential for energy generation in every cell. While our bodies naturally produce CoQ10, the concentration is higher in cells with elevated energy demands, with the heart being a prime example. As a key player in the antioxidant game, CoQ10's significance extends beyond cardiac health to encompass cellular energy, cognitive function, mitochondrial activity, and nerve well-being.

The NQ01 gene takes center stage in this intricate dance of energy transformation. Encoding the enzyme responsible for converting the oxidized form of CoQ10 (ubiquinone) into its active reduced form (ubiquinol), the NQ01 gene ensures a seamless transition. However, a Single Nucleotide Polymorphism (SNP) in this gene results in an enzyme variant with minimal capacity to convert ubiquinone to ubiquinol.

Dietary Recommendations for NQ01 Gene

Recognizing the pivotal role of NQ01, recommend dietary supplementation for all customers with this gene in their panel. The severity of the gene's impact is categorized into "Green," "Yellow," and "Red" results, each dictating a tailored approach to CoQ10 supplementation.

- **GREEN RESULT:** Supplement with 50 mg of ubiquinone. (No Variants)
- **YELLOW RESULT:** Combine 25 mg of ubiquinone with 25 mg of ubiquinol. (Single Variant)
- **RED RESULT:** Opt for 50 mg of ubiquinol exclusively. (Double Copy or two Variants)

These recommendations align with the understanding that individuals with an SNP in the NQ01 gene can derive substantial benefits from ubiquinol supplementation, the readily bioavailable form of CoQ10. Ubiquinol's support extends to optimal energy levels, cardiovascular health, and a healthy response to oxidation, making it a crucial addition to the dietary regimen, particularly for those with a compromised NQ01 gene. As our internal production of CoQ10 wanes with age, such strategic supplementation becomes increasingly relevant for overall health and well-being.

The gene NQ01_rs1800566 has been associated with an elevated susceptibility to cancer. Genetic mutations in this gene may lead to a reduced production of CoQ10, an intrinsic antioxidant present in cells and tissues throughout the body. Individuals carrying mutations in their NQ01_rs1800566 gene may face an increased likelihood of developing specific cancer types, including bladder cancer, breast cancer, colorectal cancer, and prostate cancer. It is crucial for those with such genetic mutations to engage in discussions with a healthcare professional about their cancer risk factors and collaborate on strategies to mitigate this risk. This may involve regular screenings and adopting measures to avoid environmental risks. Additionally, it's noteworthy that as we age, the internal production of CoQ10 decreases, making it especially vital for cells requiring heightened energy levels, such as those in the heart

PON1_RS662* (PARAOXONASE-1) - LIPID OXIDATION SUPPORT

What is the function of the PON-1 gene?

The PON1 gene plays a vital role in supporting healthy lipid levels and cardiovascular well-being by encoding the PON1 enzyme.

Why is the PON-1 gene significant?

The PON1 enzyme is transported on High-Density Lipoprotein (HDL) in the plasma. By binding to HDL, the PON1 enzyme shields Low-Density Lipoprotein (LDL) from oxidation. Preventing LDL oxidation is crucial, as oxidized LDL is recognized by the body as foreign, highlighting the importance of managing oxidized LDL levels for optimal cardiovascular health.

Dietary Recommendations for the PON-1 gene

The PON1 Single Nucleotide Polymorphism (SNP) is supported by ingredients that contribute to maintaining healthy lipid levels, regulating PON1 activity, and promoting overall cardiovascular health.

Mushroom Extracts (Polysaccharides):

- Reishi mushroom, with documented compounds supporting healthy lipid levels in animals.
- Similar beneficial effects are observed with Maitake and Shiitake mushrooms.

Ubiquinone and Ubiquinol:

- Green: 50 mg ubiquinone (no variants)
- Yellow: 25 mg ubiquinone and 25 mg ubiquinol (one variant)
- Red: 50 mg ubiquinol (Double copy or two variants)

Individuals with a SNP in the PON1 gene may find supplementation with ubiquinol, the bioavailable form of CoQ10, advantageous. Ubiquinol supports optimal energy, cardiovascular health, and a healthy response to oxidation.

Emphasizing lifestyle choices remains crucial, even in the presence of a minimal genetic risk. Prioritize a nutrient-rich diet centered around whole foods, including leafy green vegetables, fresh fruits, and lean proteins. Aim for regular exercise, committing to at least 5 days per week, incorporating a mix of aerobic workouts, resistance training, and flexibility exercises lasting 20-30 minutes each. Cultivate stress-relieving habits like meditation or tai chi to promote overall well-being.

IL6_RS1800795* (INTERLEUKIN 6) - HEALTHY IMMUNE SYSTEM

Interleukin 6 is a cytokine involved in the regulation of the immune system and inflammation. The rs1800795 variant is associated with differences in IL-6 production.

A healthy immune system is crucial for overall well-being, and IL-6 plays a role in immune response and inflammation. However, caring for your immune system involves various factors beyond a single genetic variant. Here are some general tips for maintaining a healthy immune system:

- **BALANCED DIET:** Consume a well-balanced diet rich in fruits, vegetables, whole grains, lean proteins, and healthy fats.

Nutrients such as vitamins C and D, zinc, and antioxidants support immune function.

- **REGULAR EXERCISE:** Engage in regular physical activity, as it helps boost the immune system and promotes overall health.

- **ADEQUATE SLEEP:** Ensure you get enough quality sleep, as sleep is essential for immune function and overall well-being.

- **STRESS MANAGEMENT:** Chronic stress can negatively impact the immune system. Practice stress-reducing activities such as meditation, yoga, or deep breathing exercises.

- **HYDRATION:** Stay hydrated, as water is essential for many bodily functions, including immune system function.

- **GOOD HYGIENE PRACTICES:** Practice good hygiene to prevent infections. This includes regular handwashing, proper food handling, and avoiding contact with sick individuals.

- **AVOID SMOKING AND EXCESSIVE ALCOHOL:** Smoking and excessive alcohol consumption can weaken the immune system. Minimize or avoid these habits for better immune health.

Dietary recommendations for IL6 gene

Turmeric Root Powder:

- Turmeric, containing the curcuminoid compound curcumin, is renowned for its anti-inflammatory properties and antioxidant benefits.

- Curcumin in turmeric inhibits NF-kB, a nuclear transcription factor that regulates the expression of genes involved in the inflammatory response.

Turmeric root powder has shown to have anti-inflammatory properties. This spice, commonly used in Indian cuisine, contains curcumin which is known for its antioxidant effects. Curcumin has been found to inhibit NF-kB, a protein complex that regulates the expression of genes involved in the inflammatory response. Adding turmeric root powder to your meals or taking it as a supplement may help reduce inflammation and promote better immune health.

A mediterranean diet is key with olive oils, wild-caught fish, and organic grass fed meat is key. NO dairy, NO wheat, NO grains, NO barley beer (rice beer if drinking). Use ginger and cinnamon, too.

It's important to note that genetic variations, like IL6_rs1800795, contribute to individual differences, but lifestyle factors also play a significant role in overall immune system function. If you have specific concerns about your genetic profile or immune health, consulting with a healthcare professional or a genetic counselor would be advisable.

TNF-A_RS1800629* (TUMOR NECROSIS FACTOR-ALPHA)

This is another gene that has been linked to immune response. Certain variations in this gene have been associated with increased susceptibility to inflammatory diseases and infections. However, maintaining a healthy lifestyle can help mitigate these genetic risks.

EXERCISE REGULARLY: While regular exercise may not prevent you from getting sick, it can boost your overall immunity by increasing the production of white blood cells and antibodies. It can also help improve your mood and reduce stress levels, which are both important for a strong immune system.

GET ENOUGH SLEEP: Lack of sleep has been shown to decrease immune function and increase susceptibility to illness. Aim for 7-8 hours of quality sleep each night to give your body time to repair and recharge.

REDUCE STRESS: Chronic stress leads to an elevated level of cortisol, a hormone that suppresses the immune system. Find healthy ways to cope with stress, such as meditation, exercise, or spending time in nature.

EAT A BALANCED DIET: A nutrient-rich diet is crucial for a strong immune system. Make sure to include plenty of fruits, vegetables, whole grains, and lean proteins in your meals. These foods provide essential vitamins and minerals that support your body's defense against illness.

STAY HYDRATED: Drinking enough water is vital for maintaining a healthy immune system. Water helps flush toxins from the body and keeps cells functioning properly. Aim for 8 glasses of water per day and avoid sugary beverages that can weaken immunity.

PRACTICE GOOD HYGIENE: Proper hygiene practices, such as washing your hands regularly and covering your mouth when coughing or sneezing, can prevent the spread of germs and viruses. Keep hand sanitizer with you for times when soap and water are not available.

STAY ACTIVE: Regular physical activity is essential for a strong immune system. Exercise helps boost circulation and supports the production of infection-fighting white blood cells. Aim for at least 30 minutes of moderate exercise each day.

GET VACCINATED: Talk to your doctor about recommended vaccinations for you and your family. Vaccines can protect against a variety of illnesses, including the flu, measles, and pneumonia. Be sure these DO NOT interfere with any other gene variant.

AVOID CLOSE CONTACT WITH SICK INDIVIDUALS: If someone around you is sick, try to limit your contact with them. This can help prevent the spread of illness to yourself and others.

AVOID TOBACCO AND EXCESS ALCOHOL: Both tobacco use and excessive alcohol consumption can weaken the immune system and increase the risk of infections. If you

GET ENOUGH VITAMIN D: Vitamin D plays an important role in immune function. Make sure to get enough sunlight exposure or take a supplement if you live in an area with limited sunlight.

Incorporating lean proteins and healthy fats into your diet can also help boost your immune system. Lean proteins such as chicken, fish, and beans provide essential amino acids that are necessary for building and repairing cells. Healthy fats found in avocados, nuts, and olive oil can help reduce inflammation and support the production of white blood cells.

Dietary guidelines for TNF-a gene

The TNF-a SNP is reinforced by ingredients specifically designed to regulate TNF-a levels, foster a balanced inflammatory response, and combat the heightened production of free radicals associated with elevated TNF-a levels and aging.

Polyphenols from Green Tea, Grape Seed, and Pomegranate Extracts:

- Increased polyphenol intake contributes to overall health and promotes healthy aging.
- Green Tea polyphenols, demonstrated in in vitro and animal studies, effectively reduce TNF-a expression.

- Human studies show that Green Tea extract supplementation lowers TNF-a levels.

- Green Tea and Grape Seed polyphenols exhibit the ability to modulate inflammatory responses in humans.

- Pomegranate polyphenols support the modulation of inflammatory cell signaling by suppressing TNF-a induction of various inflammatory proteins.

- Grape Seed extract, containing proanthocyanidins or OPCs, aids in reducing the expression of the vascular cell adhesion molecule-1 gene (VCAM-1), a key player in healthy inflammatory responses induced by TNF-a.

Milk Thistle Extract (Silymarin):

- Silymarin reduces TNF-a induced activation of NF-kB, a nuclear transcription factor regulating gene expression in the inflammatory response.

- Silymarin safeguards against TNF-a induced production of reactive oxygen species in lipid peroxidation.

- Animal studies demonstrate Silymarin's capacity to inhibit TNF-a gene expression.

Individuals with a SNP in the TNF-a gene can find valuable support through supplementation with ingredients that:

- Inhibit TNF-a activity.

- Counteract the increased production of free radicals induced by elevated TNF-a.

- Foster a balanced and healthy inflammatory response.

NOTE: *Higher levels of unhealthy inflammation show up in Rheumatoid arthritis, infection and negatively affect cells and organs with this group. There is an intestinal response with any type of food if not supported properly. Tumors, bone problems, and cancers are more likely to develop.*

GSTP1_RS1695* (GLUTATHIONE S-TRANSFERASE P1) - OXIDATIVE STRESS SUPPORT: THE ROLE OF THE GSTP1 GENE IN DETOXIFICATION:

GSTP1, part of the glutathione S-transferases family, represents a group of enzymes present in various cells.

Why is this gene critical?

These enzymes play a pivotal role in the detoxification process known as phase II detoxification. In this process, reduced glutathione binds to foreign compounds, rendering them more water-soluble. Glutathione, the most potent antioxidant in human cells, operates independently on intracellular reactive oxygen species but collaborates with GSTP1 to neutralize foreign compounds. This conjugated compound becomes non-toxic and can be expelled from the body, effectively reducing oxidative stress.

The SNP we examine leads to decreased GSTP1 protein activity, rendering cells more susceptible to oxidative stress.

Dietary Recommendations for GSTP1 gene

Broccoli Powder:

- Naturally rich in vital nutrients such as flavonoids, carotenoids, tocopherols, beta-carotene, indoles, and isothiocyanates, broccoli boasts high antioxidant properties.

Quercetin – 98%:

- An antioxidant that scavenges free radicals, quercetin also exhibits anti-inflammatory and antihistamine effects.

Resveratrol – 50%:

- A natural phenol with antioxidant properties, resveratrol contributes to the body's defense against oxidative stress.

S-Acetyl Glutathione:

- Glutathione, considered one of the body's most powerful antioxidants, provides robust support.

VDR_RS2228570* (VITAMIN D RECEPTOR)

Unlocking the Power of the VDR Gene: Harnessing Vitamin D for Optimal Bone Health

The VDR gene, also known as the Vitamin D Receptor, holds the key to effectively utilizing Vitamin D in our bodies. But why is this gene so important?

In the quest for healthy bones, Vitamin D has always been a crucial nutrient. Traditionally, we've relied on sunlight to provide us with enough Vitamin D. However, as awareness of sun damage grows and sunblock becomes more common, our ability to obtain sufficient Vitamin D from sunlight has been compromised.

Vitamin D works hand in hand with Vitamin K2 and Calcium to optimize bone density. Our bodies constantly create new bone while breaking down old bone. This delicate balance continues until around age 30, when bone resorption begins to surpass bone formation. Vitamin D plays a crucial role in maintaining calcium balance by promoting absorption in the intestines. This, in turn, promotes bone formation and allows our bodies to properly regulate calcium levels.

But that's not all. Recent evidence has shown that Vitamin D has a far-reaching impact on our overall health. It plays a role in parathyroid hormone synthesis, it modulates the endocrine and immune systems, and it even affects cardiovascular health and brain function. The current recommended intake allowance set by the government may be too low, failing to address these other vital functions of Vitamin D.

For individuals with a SNP in the VDR gene, supplementation is key. By promoting optimal calcium absorption, supporting healthy bone mineral density, and overall bone health, you can unlock the full potential of the VDR gene.

Get the most out of your bones with these dietary recommendations:

- **SPEND TIME IN THE SUNLIGHT:** 10-15 minutes per day in direct sunlight without sunscreen. Avoid prolonged time in the sun or sunburns. Eat more vitamin D rich foods: wild-caught fatty fish such as salmon, sardines, herring, and mackerel. Oats, mushrooms, and eggs are also rich in vitamin D.

- **CALCIUM (AS CALCIUM CARBONATE):** crucial for bone health.

- **VITAMIN K2** (as menaquinone): found in animal and fermented foods, essential for bone health.

- **VITAMIN D3 (AS CHOLECALCIFEROL):** necessary for maximizing calcium absorption, higher doses recommended.

Don't let your bones suffer. Harness the power of the VDR gene and take control of your bone health.

EPHX1_RS1051740* (MICROSOMAL EPOXIDE HYDROLASE) YOUR GUIDE TO HEALTHY DETOXIFICATION

Discover your genetic risk for unhealthy detoxification with the EPHX1 gene.

Here are some recommendations to maintain optimal health:

EAT A NUTRIENT-DENSE DIET: Focus on whole foods, especially green leafy vegetables and organic berries. Stay active: Exercise for at least 20-30 minutes per day, for at least 3 days a week.

Let's dive deeper into the EPHX1 gene

The EPHX1 gene plays a vital role in detoxifying harmful substances like cigarette smoke, car exhaust, pesticides, alcohol, and more. It produces the EPHX1 enzyme, which helps eliminate these toxins from the body.

Why does the EPHX1 gene matter?

Detoxification is the removal of toxic substances from the body. The liver serves as the body's first line of defense against these foreign chemicals. When the liver detoxifies these substances, it forms highly-reactive epoxides that can damage DNA and proteins. The EPHX1 enzyme helps eliminate these harmful epoxides. A poorly functioning detoxification system can impact energy levels, appetite, skin health, and stress response.

Here are a few "diet tips" for the EPHX1 gene:

Support your EPHX1 gene with the right ingredients:

1. **GREEN TEA EXTRACT:** Boosts the EPHX1 enzyme activity and supports liver health.

2. **MILK THISTLE EXTRACT:** Protects the liver against free radicals and enhances detoxification.

3. **ARTICHOKE EXTRACT:** Improves bile flow, crucial for removing toxins.

4. **CRUCIFEROUS VEGETABLES (BROCCOLI AND KALE):** Stimulate detoxification enzymes and promote toxin elimination.

5. **BURDOCK ROOT POWDER, SCHISANDRA BERRY POWDER, AND GOTU KOLA HERB EXTRACT:** Further support liver health and natural detoxification.

Living with the EPHX1 variant gene

If you have the EPHX1 variant gene, you may be at an elevated risk for heart disease and metabolic disorders due to decreased fat breakdown enzymes. Avoid environmental triggers like cigarette smoke, car exhaust, pesticides, and wood smoke. It's also best to avoid Tylenol-type products.

Making positive lifestyle changes can reduce your risk:

1. Eat a healthy diet: Focus on fiber, lean proteins, fruits, and vegetables. Limit saturated fats, cholesterol, processed foods, sugar, and refined carbs. Avoid GMO foods.

2. Stay active: Exercise regularly for at least 20-30 minutes per day, 3 times a week.

3. Manage stress and get enough rest.

4. Avoid excessive alcohol consumption, smoking, and illegal drugs.

5. Use green decaf tea and herbal supplements to reduce sensitivity.

Consult a doctor or genetic counselor for personalized guidance.

Take charge of your health and optimize your detoxification with the EPHX1 gene!

SOD2_RS4880* (MANGANESE SUPEROXIDE DISMUTASE)

Protect your body: understanding the importance of the SOD2 gene

The SOD2 gene, also known as Manganese Superoxide Dismutase, plays a crucial role in safeguarding your body against oxidation. By regulating the production of an enzyme called manganese superoxide dismutase (mSOD), this gene helps eliminate toxic superoxide free radicals that can cause damage to your cell machinery and DNA.

Why is the SOD2 gene so important? The superoxide radical, a highly toxic free radical, is present in every cell of our bodies. It can initiate damaging chain reactions, leading to the gradual wear and tear of our critical tissues. However, most organisms, including humans, have evolved an enzyme to neutralize these radicals. mSOD acts as the first line of defense against oxidative damage, effectively scavenging superoxide radicals and rendering them harmless.

To support the SOD2 gene, incorporating certain dietary recommendations can be beneficial. Antioxidant ingredients that combat the superoxide radical and increase mSOD activity are recommended. Some examples of such ingredients include:

1. **GREEN TEA AND WHITE TEA EXTRACTS:** These teas contain polyphenols and catechins that exhibit potent antioxidant properties. Epidemiological studies, cellular research, and animal studies have supported their ability to scavenge superoxide radicals and promote mSOD activity.

2. **BILBERRY EXTRACT:** The anthocyanins found in bilberry have been shown to have superoxide scavenging activity. Bilberry has traditionally been used for age-related vision problems, and it is believed this effect is due to its ability to counteract retinal oxidation damage associated with reduced mSOD.

3. **SPIRULINA POWDER:** Spirulina is rich in superoxide dismutase (mSOD) and contains phycocyanin, a plant pigment that has been found to decrease cardiac production of superoxide radicals in animal studies.

4. **NIACIN (VITAMIN B3):** Nicotinamide, a derivative of niacin, is necessary for the production of coenzymes essential for the proper functioning of mSOD.

Individuals with a SNP in the SOD2 gene can benefit from incorporating these ingredients into their supplementation regimen. These ingredients not only provide antioxidant support but also help manage all free radicals and promote a healthy response to oxidation.

To fully support this genetic variant, it is essential to make lifestyle changes. Incorporating a balanced diet with an emphasis on fruits and vegetables, regular exercise, stress management, and avoiding smoking can significantly reduce the risk of serious diseases.

Remember, the choices you make regarding your lifestyle today can have a positive impact on your overall health in the future. Prioritize your well-being and steer clear of toxic relationships that can create additional cell damage. Opt for a plastic-free lifestyle and avoid reheating or cooking food in plastic containers. To further support your SOD2 gene, aim to eat more colorful foods, exercise regularly, and consider detox methods like infrared sauna or hot yoga to eliminate toxins. Limit alcohol consumption and steer clear of processed breads and dyes.

Regular blood work with your healthcare provider can help monitor your progress and ensure your body is in optimal condition. Take charge of your health and protect your body by understanding the importance of the SOD2 gene.

FUT2_RS602662* (GALACTOSIDE 2-ALPHA-L-FUCOSYLTRANSFERASE 2) - VITAMIN B12

Unlock the Secret to Optimal Health with the FUT2 Gene!

Discover the vital role of the FUT2 gene in maintaining a healthy gut microbiome and optimizing vitamin B12 absorption. This gene is responsible for cultivating beneficial bacteria in the gut, which is essential for overall well-being. Without a healthy microbiome, our bodies struggle to absorb vitamin B12, which can lead to a host of health issues.

Nourish your gut for maximum benefits!

This gene is responsible for producing the good bacteria that are essential for our overall health. When your gut is teeming with beneficial bacteria, it creates an environment that allows vitamin B12 to be properly absorbed and utilized by your body. However, an unhealthy gut can hinder this process and deprive you of the countless benefits of vitamin B12.

To ensure your FUT2 gene functions at its best, nourish your gut with the right foods and supplements. Incorporate nutrient-rich mushrooms, algae, oats, and barley into your diet. Avoid processed, fried, and sugary foods as much as possible. Say goodbye to afternoon fatigue and welcome vibrant energy!

Don't let bad bacteria take over!

People with lower B12 levels may experience anemia, impaired immune function, and the proliferation of harmful bacteria. Combat this by adding prebiotic-rich foods such as garlic, onions, leeks, asparagus, and apples to your daily meals. AVOID keto or carnivore diets.

*Exercise 3x week 20-30 minutes.

Take control of your gut health and unlock the full potential of your FUT2 gene. With the right approach, you can improve your overall well-being and enrich your life.

Talk to your doctor about methylated B12 supplementation.

FTO_RS9939609* (ALPHA-KETOGLUTARATE-DEPENDENT DIOXYGENASE FTO) - HEALTHY WEIGHT MANAGEMENT

It's important to maintain a healthy lifestyle. Follow a nutrient-dense diet with plenty of green leafy vegetables and organic berries, and make exercise a priority by committing to 20-30 minutes of physical activity at least three days a week.* Avoid excessive sugar intake.

The FTO gene, also known as fat mass and obesity associated protein, plays a role in weight regulation. Common variants of this gene have been associated with obesity, increased body mass index (BMI), and higher calorie consumption. FTO gene variants are also linked to type II diabetes and metabolic syndrome. While the exact mechanism is still being studied, it's clear that the FTO gene is involved in obesity.

For individuals with an FTO gene variant, consider incorporating the following into your diet to support healthy weight management:

- Berberine, a bioactive alkaloid, helps regulate metabolism.

- Vitamin C is associated with body fat oxidation and lower BMI.

- Alpha Lipoic Acid can decrease blood sugar levels and restore vitamin levels.

If you have the FTO variant, you may have a tendency to hold on to sugars and fat, which can lead to obesity and metabolic disorders. It's important to make lasting changes to your diet and exercise routine to reduce the risk. A balanced diet, regular physical activity, and monitoring by your doctor can help maintain a healthy weight and manage cholesterol and blood pressure levels.

To support your health, focus on a Mediterranean diet, intermittent fasting with protein-rich meals, and smaller portion sizes throughout the day. Avoid high glycemic foods, processed foods, starchy breads, and sugary condiments. Incorporate dark, leafy green vegetables and healthy fats into your meals. Be mindful of product ingredients when making purchases.

Take control of your health and make informed choices to support a healthy weight and overall well-being.

Take control of your heart health today!

Know where your DNA weaknesses and strengths are!

DNA GROUPINGS

NAME_____ DATE _____

HEART

ENERGY

GUT

BRAIN

DETOX

IMMUNE/
INFLAMMATION

CHAPTER 12
DNA GROUPINGS

Your DNA genes are broken down into groupings. What does this mean? It means that each person's DNA contains certain combinations of genes that are unique to them. These groupings can tell us a lot about our health, ancestry, and even some traits we may have inherited from our ancestors. Knowing your DNA groupings is important for understanding how diet, lifestyle habits, and environment can affect your individual health needs.

You can access the grouping chart here: https://drive.google.com/file/d/1lIWz1Yh1KkEWZkxOWcJgW_xEXwIE5GQc/view?usp=sharing

There are six groupings or filters which the gene variants are applied to.

HEART

- ApoB_rs693* (Apolipoprotein B)
- CYP11B2_rs1799998* (Aldosterone Synthase)
- MTHFR_rs1801133* (Methylene Tetrahydrofolate Reductase)
- MTHFR_rs1801131* (Methylene Tetrahydrofolate Reductase)

- MTRR_rs1801394* (Methionine Synthase Reductase)
- NQ01_rs1800566* (Coenzyme Q10 Reductase)
- PON1_rs662* (Paraoxonase-1)

IMMUNE/INFLAMMATION

- CRP_rs1205* (C-reactive Protein)
- IL6_rs1800795* (Interleukin 6)
- MTHFR_rs1801133* (Methylene Tetrahydrofolate Reductase)
- MTHFR_rs1801131* (Methylene Tetrahydrofolate Reductase)
- MTRR_rs1801394* (Methionine Synthase Reductase)
- TNF-a_rs1800629* (Tumor Necrosis Factor-alpha)
- GSTP1_rs1695* (Glutathione S-transferase P1)
- VDR_rs2228570* (Vitamin D Receptor)

ENERGY

- ATP5C1_rs1244414* Mitochondrial ATP Synthase
- EPHX1_rs1051740* (Microsomal Epoxide Hydrolase)
- MTHFR_rs1801133* (Methylene Tetrahydrofolate Reductase)
- MTHFR_rs1801131* (Methylene Tetrahydrofolate Reductase)
- NQ01_rs1800566* (Coenzyme Q10 Reductase)
- SOD2_rs4880* (Manganese Superoxide Dismutase)
- VDR_rs2228570* (Vitamin D Receptor)

DETOX

- EPHX1_rs1051740* (Microsomal Epoxide Hydrolase)
- GSTP1_rs1695* (Glutathione S-transferase P1)
- MTHFR_rs1801133* (Methylene Tetrahydrofolate Reductase)
- MTHFR_rs1801131* (Methylene Tetrahydrofolate Reductase)
- SOD2_rs4880* (Manganese Superoxide Dismutase)

BRAIN

- ATP5C1_rs1244414* Mitochondrial ATP Synthase
- FUT2_rs602662* (Galactoside 2-alpha-L-fucosyltransferase 2)
- GSTP1_rs1695* (Glutathione S-transferase P1)
- MTHFR_rs1801133* (Methylene Tetrahydrofolate Reductase)
- MTHFR_rs1801131* (Methylene Tetrahydrofolate Reductase)
- NQ01_rs1800566* (Coenzyme Q10 Reductase)
- SOD2_rs4880* (Manganese Superoxide Dismutase)
- VDR_rs2228570* (Vitamin D Receptor)

GUT

- FUT2_rs602662* (Galactoside 2-alpha-L-fucosyltransferase 2)
- GSTP1_rs1695* (Glutathione S-transferase P1)
- MTHFR_rs1801133* (Methylene Tetrahydrofolate Reductase)
- MTHFR_rs1801131* (Methylene Tetrahydrofolate Reductase)
- VDR_rs2228570* (Vitamin D Receptor)

Knowing the DNA combinations and how they affect your body can help you make decisions about your diet and lifestyle so that you can live a healthier life. Knowing how certain genes affect your body can help you create more targeted nutrition and exercise plans that meet your specific needs. If a person's DNA combination shows they are at risk for heart disease, then they may want to focus on eating foods that are heart-healthy and exercising regularly. Or, if a person has an immune/inflammation DNA variant, they may want to focus on taking supplements that support their immune system and reducing inflammation in their diet.

By understanding your unique genetic makeup, you can tailor your nutrition and lifestyle choices to maximize your health potential. Your journey to better health begins with knowing the six DNA groupings that affect nutrition and exercise. Once you identify your type, you'll be able to make lifestyle changes to improve your overall health.

With the right information, you can unlock the power of your genetic code to achieve better health. With DNA-based nutrition and exercise plans, you can become a healthier version of yourself!

Your genetics don't have to be a roadblock to living a long, healthy life. With the right guidance and nutrition plan, you can maximize your health potential based on your individual needs. Working with a certified genetic professional is the best way to get personalized advice that fits your unique genetic makeup.

By understanding your genetics and tailoring your diet and lifestyle accordingly, you can enjoy a healthier life for years to come. With the right information and plan, you can turn your genetic code into an asset!

The power of understanding your genetic profile can help improve your overall health. Start on the path to better health today with a comprehensive genetic analysis and personalized advice. Unlock the potential of your genetic code for a healthier lifestyle now!

By following an individualized nutrition plan designed for your unique genetic profile, you can feel confident that your health is in the right hands. Knowing your genetic predisposition to certain conditions and diseases will help you make informed decisions that may significantly improve your overall wellbeing.

It's never been easier to take charge of your future health! With a simple swab test, you can unlock the power of genetics and finally take control of your health. Get started on the path to better health today with an easy-to-understand, comprehensive genetic analysis and personalized advice tailored to you.

Know your DNA,
Know your health!

Need more information? Check out these 2 game changing videos.

https://V8554044.nucleogenexmsg.com/kaIFvkXmjO?Method=C

https://V8554044.nucleogenexmsg.com/325t31uSv1?Method=C

YourDailyNourishment

"A good beginning makes a good ending."

CHAPTER 13

THE EPILOGUE

Family—the dynamics can change at any time, without notice. I grew up with one sister who was very special to me growing up. We were totally different as many siblings can be. Our parents kept us close to family, enough that we knew all of our cousins on both sides. Most weekends and summer vacations were spent with extended family. So family has a special place in my heart.

So many of us never have the opportunity to meet and know and learn from our extended family. We are born in completely different times, with different lifestyles and opportunities available. That doesn't mean that we don't have to rely on our families for guidance in this modern world. It wasn't until my mom passed away that I had the opportunity to learn more about her childhood from a cousin who grew up very close to her.

For many years I wondered why mom was so strong-willed, yet you could feel and see her heart was empty and there was a yearning for love and compassion. It was through the stories of her childhood that I realized why. Family, in all its forms, is important to our identity and understanding. It's difficult for us to go out into the world without knowing about those who came before us.

Shortly after I was married and on Thanksgiving, I received a phone call from a woman who had been adopted and through her research had found her birth mother. Yes, we shared the same mother. My husband and I were both taken back by this and were not certain what to think.

At our first meeting there was not a doubt we were sisters. As I got to know my newfound sister, we discovered that we shared many similarities: similar interests, looks and especially the love of dancing. Years later, we found there was an older sister who had also been given up for adoption. They both want and need to know what DNA predispositions run in the family. It is so wonderful to have them both in my life.

But wait! Here is the curve ball! Over the years, through DNA ancestry testing, I found out that the father I grew up with was not my biological father. New family members started to emerge, and over the next few decades, I found I had seven half-siblings. I have met all but one brother.

What have I learned from this? Take time to learn from your family members, no matter how old or close they are. Hear their stories and let them know you cherish what they have to say so they will keep sharing with you. Celebrate your heritage by learning more about the people you are connected to; it can be rewarding! Don't take for granted the knowledge that lies within your family tree. It's yours for a lifetime!

We all face similar challenges and seek to make sense of their reality. It can be difficult to navigate through the ever-changing landscape of illnesses, technology, medical advances, privacy laws, etc., but it is possible! Whether you're looking into genetic testing because you don't know where you came from, you were adopted, carrier screening or medical research; learning about your family history; or trying to figure out how or when to share sensitive data with your family members, you can trust that there are professionals available to help you understand every step of the way. With the right resources and expertise, you can form a stronger bond with those around you.

Be sure to keep a log or record of your family's history that is accurately documented so that it can be enjoyed for generations to come. It will help you connect your past with your future!

The advent of advanced DNA testing technologies has brought both incredible insights and ethical challenges to the forefront. Discrimination based on genetic markers, a concern that has escalated with the rise in popularity of personal genetic testing, poses a significant ethical dilemma.

While uncovering one's genetic predispositions can offer valuable information about health risks and ancestry, it also opens the door to potential misuse of this sensitive data. The fear is that employers, insurers, or other entities could exploit genetic information to discriminate against individuals based on their inherent characteristics, leading to unfair treatment in areas such as employment, insurance coverage, or even social interactions.

Striking a balance between the promise of genetic advancements and protecting individuals from discrimination requires robust legislation, privacy safeguards, and public awareness campaigns. The ethical considerations surrounding DNA testing underscore the need for a thoughtful and responsible approach to harnessing the power of genetic information for the betterment of individuals and society as a whole.

This book has shared my insights into the intricate interplay of our body, life, and elements, and has aimed to guide you towards conscious choices in nourishing your physical and emotional well-being. Now, as we come to the end of this journey, I want to remind you that optimal heart health goes beyond just physical health.

Maintaining a balanced diet and regular exercise are crucial for a healthy heart, gut, brain function, immune system, and energy levels. It is equally important to nourish your soul. Our emotional and mental well-being have a direct impact on our physical health, including our heart health.

To truly achieve optimal health, it is necessary to find balance in all aspects of our lives—physically, emotionally, mentally, and spiritually. This may include practicing mindfulness techniques such as meditation or journaling, surrounding yourself with positive influences and relationships, and finding activities that bring joy and fulfillment into your life.

It is also important to pay attention to the signals your body is sending you. Knowing your DNA blueprint and being aware of any potential genetic predispositions can help you make informed decisions about your lifestyle. This includes understanding your family history of heart disease and taking preventative measures if necessary.

A diet rich in whole, unprocessed foods such as fruits, vegetables, lean proteins, and healthy fats is essential for keeping our hearts functioning at their best. Avoiding excessive amounts of sugar, salt, and unhealthy fats can also lower the risk for heart disease.

Regular physical activity is also key in protecting our heart health. Engaging in moderate exercise for at least 30 minutes a day not only helps maintain a healthy weight but also strengthens the heart muscles and improves circulation. It is important to find activities that we enjoy and can incorporate into our daily routines, whether it be walking, dancing, or playing a sport.

Another factor in maintaining heart health is managing stress levels. Chronic stress can put a strain on the heart and contribute to the development of heart disease. Finding ways to relax and unwind such as meditation, yoga, or spending time outdoors can help reduce stress levels.

In addition to emotional well-being, social connections are also crucial for your health. Studies have shown that people with strong social support systems tend to have better cardiovascular health than those who feel socially isolated. This can include spending time with friends and loved ones, joining community groups or clubs, or even volunteering for a cause you care about.

In understanding the essence of well-being, consider adopting paths that secure the foundations of your health. From dietary transformations and mindset shifts to bodily examinations – when these align harmoniously, the potential for enhanced well-being becomes imminent.

May this journey leave you enriched, providing you with a new perspective on the complexities within your body. I believe that by sharing these insights, we contribute to deepening the collective understanding of the knowledge we possess in our time.

Thank you for taking the time to read about my passion. I hope it has given you the hope and knowledge you need to embark on your own journey towards well-being and extending your health-iest lifespan. Remember, the path to a healthier and happier life is not about perfection, but rather progress and self-care.

ENDORSEMENTS

When I first came across Patty's work with epigenetic testing, my mind was blown. I had no idea the impact of DNA on chronic health conditions. Patty is clearly passionate about her mission to help call awareness to epigenetic testing as a life-saving resource for those of us who suffer from mystery illnesses. Her book is a wonderful resource that sheds light on how epigenetic testing may just save your life, or the life of a loved one.

I can't recommend enough!

—NICOLLETE MOORE, Brand Strategist

Patty makes it very simple to understand Genetics.

This is a great book of her story and how learning about your health and your DNA markers can help guide you through your life...It's a must read!

To understand how our genes play a part in our future and understanding where we come from and knowing our blueprint can help us to make decisions in the future.

—LILIANA LOPEZ, Digital Creator

I highly recommend 'The DNA Advantage' to anyone interested in harnessing the power of genetics to support their health and well-being. With its accessible writing style and wealth of information, this book is a must-read for anyone seeking to unlock the secrets of their DNA and embrace a healthier future. In reading 'The DNA Advantage', I found myself researching and seeking answers for my own health.

—LOUANNE HUNT, Certified Success Coach, 2-times Best Selling Author and Host of the top 10 inspirational Podcast, The Mindset Playground

The DNA Advantage is not just a book, it's a heartfelt journey of healing, growth, and transformation. Patty Lach Daigle writes a truly remarkable book. It seamlessly blends personal health issues with valuable insights into health and wellness. Patty's own experiences serve as a powerful story. She is able to share her knowledge and give readers the tools that they need for healthier living. Whether discussing the importance of epigenetics, DNA testing, or the significance of personal growth, each chapter is explored with genuine passion that shines through. The DNA Advantage is a book that speaks to the power of resilience, gratitude, and the human spirit. I highly recommend it to anyone looking for inspiration and insight on their own path to wellness.

—DEBBIE MADIOU, President, The Network Marketing Magazine (TNWM)

ACKNOWLEDGMENTS

I want to give special thanks to my husband who supported me throughout this journey, especially during those long days when I was taking courses and researching. Your unwavering love and encouragement kept me going.

To my friend Mimi Hoff who introduced me to the world of epigenetics and mentors who helped and continue to give me confidence in my own abilities and personal growth. Your guidance and support have been invaluable.

To my clients who have trusted me to guide them on their health journey, thank you for allowing me to be a part of your transformation.

And last but not least, I dedicate this book to all those who are struggling with their health and searching for answers. May this book provide you with the knowledge and tools necessary to take control of your health and transform your life.

ABOUT THE AUTHOR

The DNA Advantage tells my inspirational story and enlightens the reader how using Epigenetic and Nutrigenomic testing has changed my life.

I was a young girl who grew up in a New Jersey coastal town with her parents and one sister, coming from a Catholic family where it was fish every Friday and pasta almost every weekend. My father was an avid fisherman, and both parents were blue collar factory workers.

After graduating high school, I knew college was not an option, but I knew I had to make a living for myself. This is when I started working at a local bowling alley. After a year of this, I knew I needed and wanted more. Riding my bike to the beach was my favorite pastime, and one day, I found myself at the military recruiting station. Three months later, I left home in September of 1977 to join the US Air Force.

Being stationed in South Carolina, Okinawa, Japan, Alaska, Washington DC area, and Virginia gave me the opportunity to see and experience different cultures. Travel became a passion. As I traveled to different countries playing varsity softball and volleyball, I also continued to expand my knowledge and skills through various courses and certifications offered by the military. I became proficient in computer systems and technology, which at the time was a relatively new field, and Contracts Management, which was my military career field.

I became a single mom at the age of 30, and more than halfway through my career, I met and married my husband of thirty years. This would be the start of many new journeys.

After serving active duty for 20 years in the Air Force, I decided it was now time to get that college degree. Working a full-time job, raising a family, and taking classes every other weekend for a year and a half was reality.

I retired at the age of 60, but had too much energy and felt unfulfilled. I was searching for my passion. It took me getting sick with what I thought had no alternatives to healing, to get me praying for a solution.

Through this journey of self-discovery and continuous learning, I have found my passion: helping others reach their full potential and achieving their dreams through DNA health.

HOW TO CONNECT WITH THE AUTHOR.

Patricia L Daigle, *Independent Nucleogenex Affiliate*

Connect for a 30 min FREE CONSULTATION: https://calendly.com/yourdailynourishment/30min

FACEBOOK: https://www.facebook.com/pldaigle3

INSTAGRAM: https://www.facebook.com/pldaigle3

YOUTUBE: www.youtube.com/@pattylachdaigle17481

LINKEDIN: https://www.linkedin.com/in/pattylachdaigle/

LANDING PAGE: https://www.aweber.com/users/landing_pages/import/ed128690-cd8a-49e2-8da9-158a273d4aa8

ORDER YOUR DNA TEST KIT & ÜTRITION:
https://nucleogenex.com/daiglep3

START YOUR OWN NUTRITIONAL GENOMICS BUSINESS:
https://mynucleogenex.com/daiglep3/join

www.ingramcontent.com/pod-product-compliance
Lightning Source LLC
Chambersburg PA
CBHW060235030426
42335CB00014B/1460